151 Skin Cases

Diagnosis and Treatment

151 Skin Cases
Diagnosis and Treatment

Third Edition

Sanjay Ghosh MD

Professor and Head of the Department
Department of Dermatology and Venereology
MGM Medical College and LSK Hospital
Kishanganj, Bihar, India
Medical Director (Honorary)
Institute of Allergic and Immunologic Skin Diseases (IAISD)
Kolkata, West Bengal, India

JAYPEE

JAYPEE BROTHERS MEDICAL PUBLISHERS

The Health Sciences Publisher
New Delhi | London | Panama

Jaypee Brothers Medical Publishers (P) Ltd

Headquarters

Jaypee Brothers Medical Publishers (P) Ltd
4838/24, Ansari Road, Daryaganj
New Delhi 110 002, India
Phone: +91-11-43574357
Fax: +91-11-43574314
Email: jaypee@jaypeebrothers.com

Overseas Offices

J.P. Medical Ltd
83 Victoria Street, London
SW1H 0HW (UK)
Phone: +44 20 3170 8910
Fax: +44 (0)20 3008 6180
Email: info@jpmedpub.com

Jaypee-Highlights Medical Publishers Inc
City of Knowledge, Bld. 235, 2nd Floor, Clayton
Panama City, Panama
Phone: +1 507-301-0496
Fax: +1 507-301-0499
Email: cservice@jphmedical.com

Jaypee Brothers Medical Publishers (P) Ltd
17/1-B Babar Road, Block-B, Shaymali
Mohammadpur, Dhaka-1207
Bangladesh
Mobile: +08801912003485
Email: jaypeedhaka@gmail.com

Jaypee Brothers Medical Publishers (P) Ltd
Bhotahity, Kathmandu, Nepal
Phone: +977-9741283608
Email: kathmandu@jaypeebrothers.com

Website: www.jaypeebrothers.com
Website: www.jaypeedigital.com

Inquiries for bulk sales may be solicited at: jaypee@jaypeebrothers.com

151 Skin Cases: Diagnosis and Treatment / **Sanjay Ghosh**

First Edition: 2005
Second Edition: 2014
Third Edition: **2019**

ISBN: 978-93-5270-492-7

Printed at

Dedicated to

My wife Shrabani

Regarding this Book

- Primary aim of this book is to judge the clinical acumen. The book, however, does not ignore the importance of investigations by laboratory and other methods, which may be necessary in many clinical situation to confirm diagnosis, assess degree of severity, and find associated features
- The target readers of this book are MBBS undergraduate students or practicing physicians who have not done any specialization in dermatology. Hence, common skin diseases have mostly been described but some uncommon and major dermatological cases signifying serious prognosis or systemic involvement demanding immediate referral have been included as well
- Treatment guidelines represent only sketchy plan to treat the individual case described which may require elaboration in certain cases and may not be applicable to all similar cases
- Only standard conventional treatment mentioned in the authentic textbooks or journals have been mentioned omitting therapies which are not much evidence-based
- Standard dose of the drugs have been mentioned which will, of course, depend on body weight, other concurrent medication, liver and renal status, known drug allergy, etc.
- Pre-therapy and post-therapy monitoring of drugs by laboratory tests should be done whenever required
- This book does not insist that all the cases should be managed by nondermatologists. The book has attempted to provide a basic visual knowledge for diagnosis of certain skin disorders along with basic management strategy for the primary-care physicians. Referral to dermatologist seems to be desirable whenever situation arises.

Preface to the Third Edition

This book was first launched 13 years back and with huge demand from medical students and practicing doctors, the second edition was introduced in 2014 with increased number and new set of cases. Day by day the book is getting more response from the readers, which encouraged me to bring again a new edition so early. This edition has not much change except addition of some new superficial fungal diseases as, in India recently, these diseases have been spreading like an epidemic and became quite refractory to treatment. To keep the size of the book concise and handy, I have not extended the number of cases rather omitted some rare cases which are not encountered in regular clinical practice. Hope this edition of the book would be similar success like the previous one.

I must give my sincere thanks to M/s Jaypee Brothers Medical Publishers (P) Ltd. for their help and cooperation for bringing out this edition of the book in daylight. I will be grateful if the readers accept this edition as a helpful weapon for combating skin problem in their day-to-day clinical practice.

I feel all my efforts would go in vain unless the readers find the book suitable for their need. Any clarification or queries may be made to me directly by e-mail (*drsanjayghosh1@gmail.com*).

Sanjay Ghosh

Preface to the First Edition

Dermatological training is often inadequately executed in MBBS undergraduate and post-MBBS internship days which leads to the qualifying remarks either 'too difficult' or 'very simple' regarding the subject 'Dermatology' by some qualified doctors in their practice. Some feel interest but are very much apprehensive about diagnosing and managing even an easy case confidently. Some consider the subject by oversimplification and diagnose each ring shaped case as a ring worm or tinea. They never find any depth in dermatology! Many others are totally indifferent about the subject. Of course, there are large numbers of physicians who, even without any specialization in the subject, have acquired the unique skill to deal skin cases adequately and confidently.

Whatever may be the attitude of the physician towards the subject, each and every doctor whether practicing or non-practicing has to face and even treat dermatological cases in certain situation. Hence, doctors should have some basic concept about the subject of dermatology so that they do not take the cases casually. They may not manage the case but they should know when to refer the patient to prevent fatality.

Another myth regarding the skin cases is that skin cases neither kill nor are cured. Yes, skin cases can cause life-threatening situations such as Stevens-Johnson syndrome (SJS), toxic epidermal necrolysis (TEN), erythroderma, drug hypersensitivity syndrome, pemphigus vulgaris, bullous pemphigoid, and malignant melanoma. Scabies, by secondary infection, may lead to acute glomerulonephritis, a fatal condition if not treated promptly. Manifestations of some of the serious systemic ailments may be first detected on skin, e.g., purpura from leukemias, nodules from metastases of internal malignancy, hyperpigmentation from Addison's disease, etc.

This book represents a small attempt to bridge the gap or a humble dialogue to communicate. This endeavor, however, has been based totally on visual language, which remains the basic conversation in clinical dermatology. However, this small book would never be able to substitute larger textbooks or atlas published earlier with the same mission and above all practical clinical training and day-to-day practice.

The book would never be written unless the continuous urge, encouragement and request of Mr Tarun Duneja, the General Manager (Publishing) of M/s Jaypee Brothers Medical Publishers (P) Ltd., New Delhi, India, the eminent medical publisher of the country, who had a long experience and association with our medical fraternity. I must give deep regards to him and his entire publishing team, both in New Delhi and Kolkata, who have supported whole-heartedly this project.

I must also give sincere thanks to Mr Tapas Kr Kayal, for doing the DTP and all laborious computer jobs for me in spite of his period of personal grief and turmoil.

I feel all my efforts would go in vain unless the readers find the book suitable for their need. Any clarification or queries may be made to me directly by e-mail (*drsanjayghosh1@gmail.com*).

Sanjay Ghosh

Contents

Case 1

A 35-year-old male had acute onset grouped painful skin vesicles, some hemorrhagic, on left side of abdomen and loin unilaterally in dermatomal distribution for last 3 days.

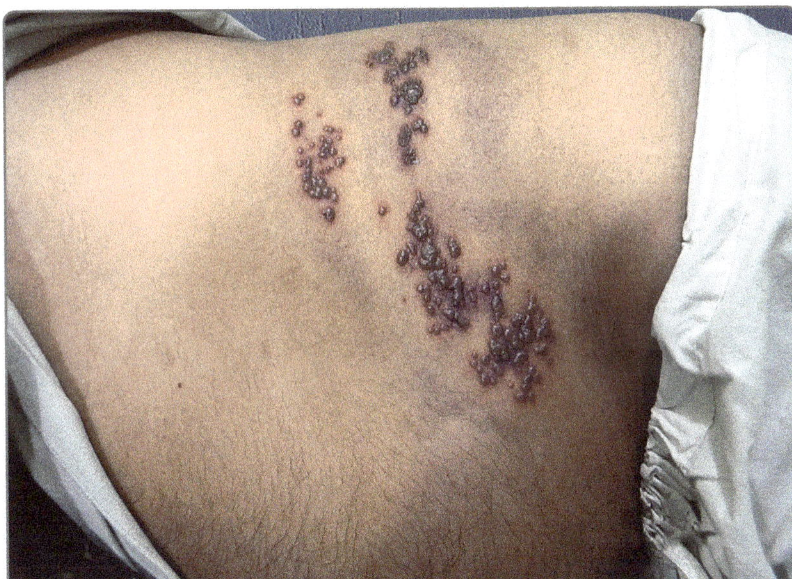

Q. What is the (i) diagnosis and (ii) management?

Answers

i. Herpes zoster.
ii. Management
  - Valacyclovir 1,000 mg 8 hourly for 7 days or acyclovir 800 mg 5 times a day for 7 days or famciclovir 500 mg 8 hourly for 7 days
  - Oral antibiotics preferably macrolides for 5–7 days to prevent secondary infection
  - Analgesic and sedatives as per need.

Case 2

A 56-year-old male had the raised skin plaque with web-like extension at the periphery on anterior chest for last about 15 years and complained of excessive itching and pain.

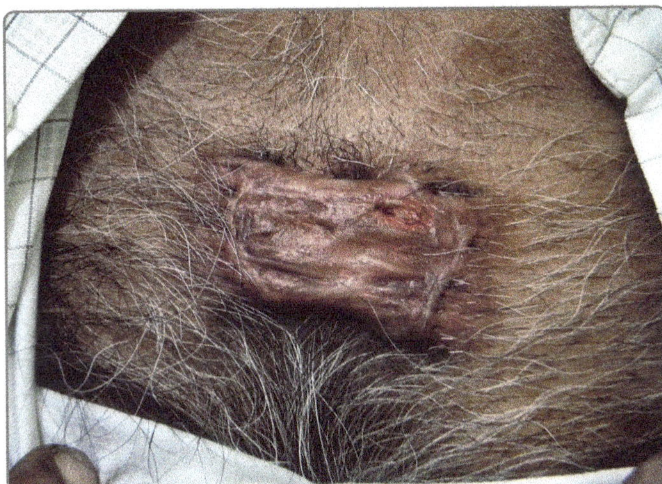

Q. What is the (i) diagnosis and (ii) management?

Answers

i. Keloid.

ii. Management
   - Intralesional triamcinolone injection (dose 10 mg/mL) with or without silicon gel sheet occlusion
   - Cryotherapy.

Case 3

A 29-year-old man had sudden onset itchy and burning vesicles and papules on right shoulder for last 2 days. The lesions were mostly distributed linearly but the papulovesicles were neither grouped in arrangement nor limited to dermatomal area.

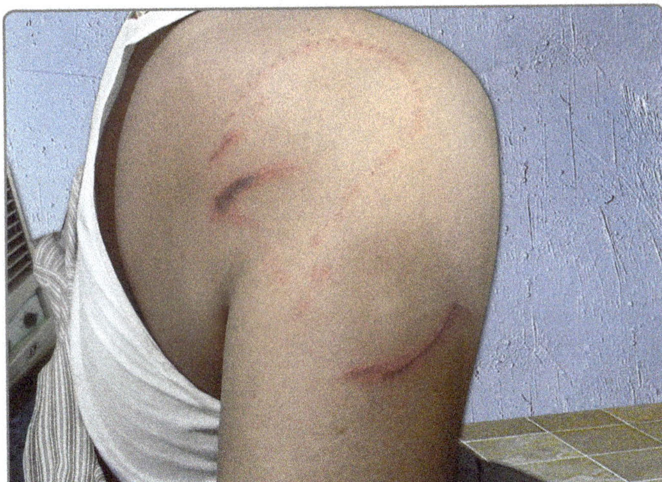

Q. What is the (i) diagnosis and (ii) management?

Answers

i. Insect hypersensitivity.

ii. Management
- Topical potent steroid lotion or cream twice daily for 1 week
- Oral antihistamines
- Oral antibiotics (short course).

Case 4

A 62-year-old lady had developed acute onset pruritic erythematous eruption with papulovesicles and oozing on dorsum of both feet for last 2 weeks after wearing a leather shoe. She had also vesicular eruption on both hands for last 1 week.

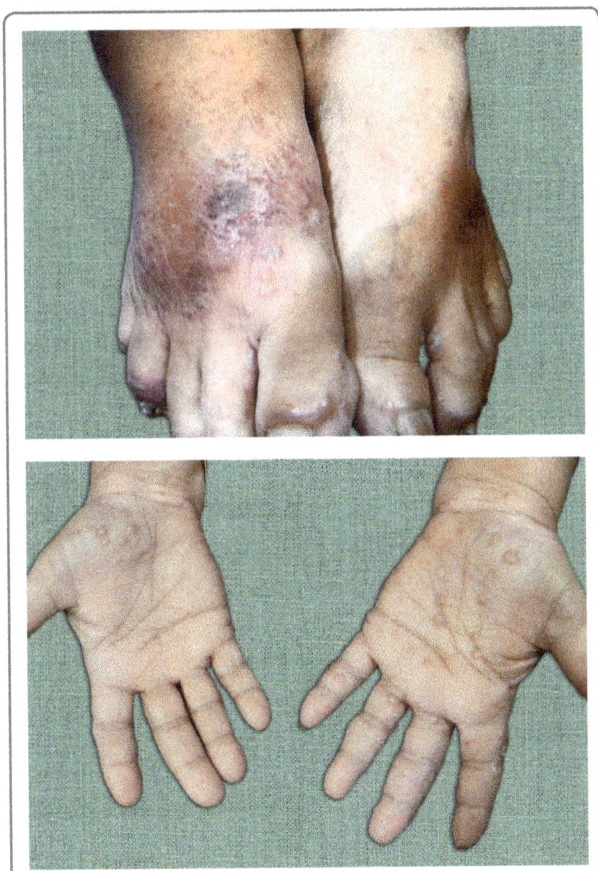

Q. What is the (i) diagnosis and (ii) management?

Answers

i. Acute contact dermatitis (feet) with id eruption (hands) [allergic contact dermatitis (ACDS) stage IIIA].

ii. Management
   - Topical corticosteroid (potent) cream on feet and hands
   - Oral antihistamines
   - Oral antibiotics (short course)
   - Oral corticosteroids (short course), if refractory
   - Allergic patch test to detect nature of footwear allergens.

Case 5

A 41-year-old lady had whitish plaque on tongue for last 2 years which can not be removed by scraping. She had also reticulated pattern of whitish eruption on her buccal mucosa for same duration.

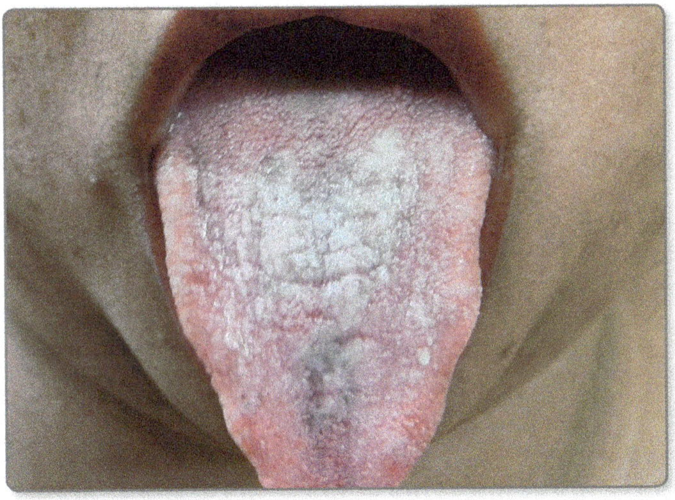

Q. What is the (i) diagnosis and (ii) management?

Answers

i. Oral lichen planus (tongue).

ii. Management

- Replacement of metal (including gold) or amalgam dental restorations, if present
- Topical corticosteroids in orabase followed by topical tacrolimus 0.1% or pimecrolimus 1%
- Topical (clotrimazole troche or mouth paint) or oral antifungal (fluconazole) to reduce secondary candida overgrowth.

Case 6

A 57-year-old male had history of non-healing ulceration on left ankle for last 1 year and on examination he had anesthesia on left leg and feet alongwith thickened left lateral popliteal nerve.

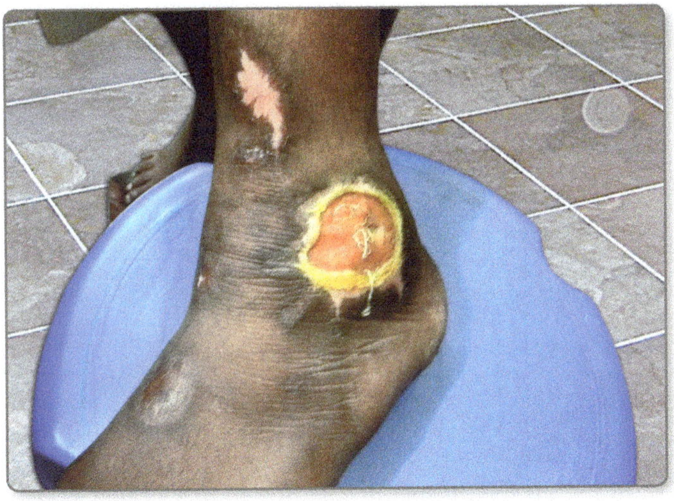

Q. What is the (i) diagnosis and (ii) management?

Answers

i. Leprosy (purely neural) with trophic ulcer.

ii. Management

- Multidrug therapy [dapsone 100 mg daily, clofazimine 50 mg daily and rifampicin 600 mg monthly (supervised)]
- Care of the ulcer: Wound swab for bacterial culture and sensitivity, normal saline wash, topical silver sulfadiazine or fucidic acid cream
- Care of the anesthetic limbs: Strict avoidance of hot contact and trauma, proper shoe (preferably microcellular rubber).

Case 7

A 33-year-old man developed sudden onset multiple dark patches upon erythematous background on back and abdomen for last 4 days. He had similar patches on the same sites 8 months back. History revealed that he had taken tinidazole preceding the eruption both the times.

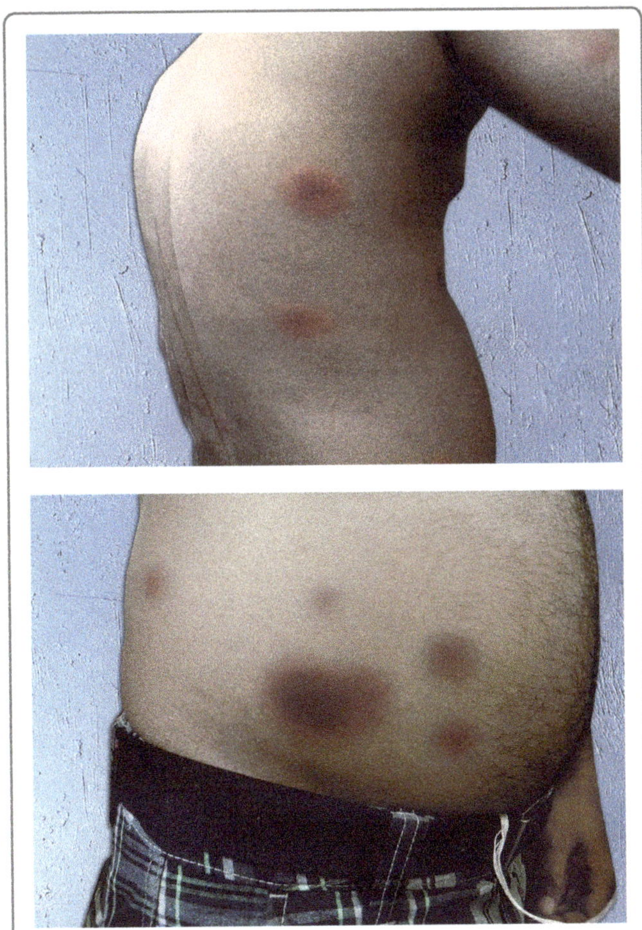

Q. What is the (i) diagnosis and (ii) management?

Answers

i. Fixed drug eruption.

ii. Management

- Strict avoidance of offending drug and cross-reacting drugs
- Topical potent steroid once daily for 3 weeks
- Oral antihistamines.

Case 8

A 31-year-lady had localized eczematous eruption on left upper eyelid only for last 2 weeks. She had history of application for last 2 months of a nail polish of new color, which she had not used before.

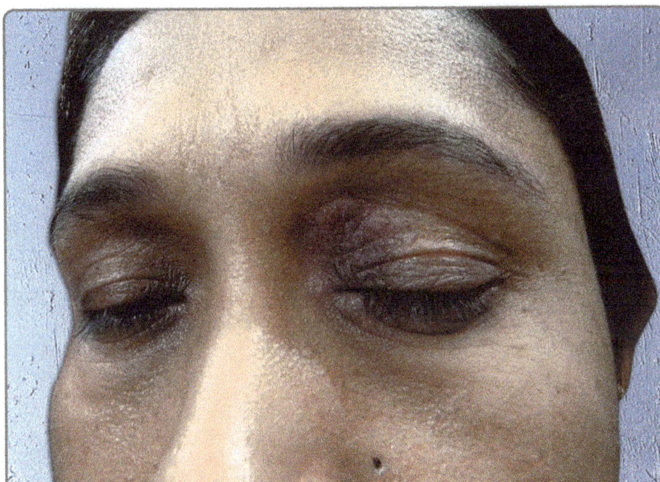

Q. What is the (i) diagnosis and (ii) management?

Answers

i. Allergic contact dermatitis (ACD) [commonest site of ACD from nail polish is eyelid, which is usually unilateral].

ii. Management
   - Strict avoidance of nail polish
   - Low potent steroid cream once daily for 7 days
   - Oral antihistamines for 7 days.

Case 9

An 18-year-old boy had pruritic multiple annular lesions with central clearing and scaly inflammed border with papulovesicles on face, lower abdomen ,and groin rapidly spreading for last 2 months.

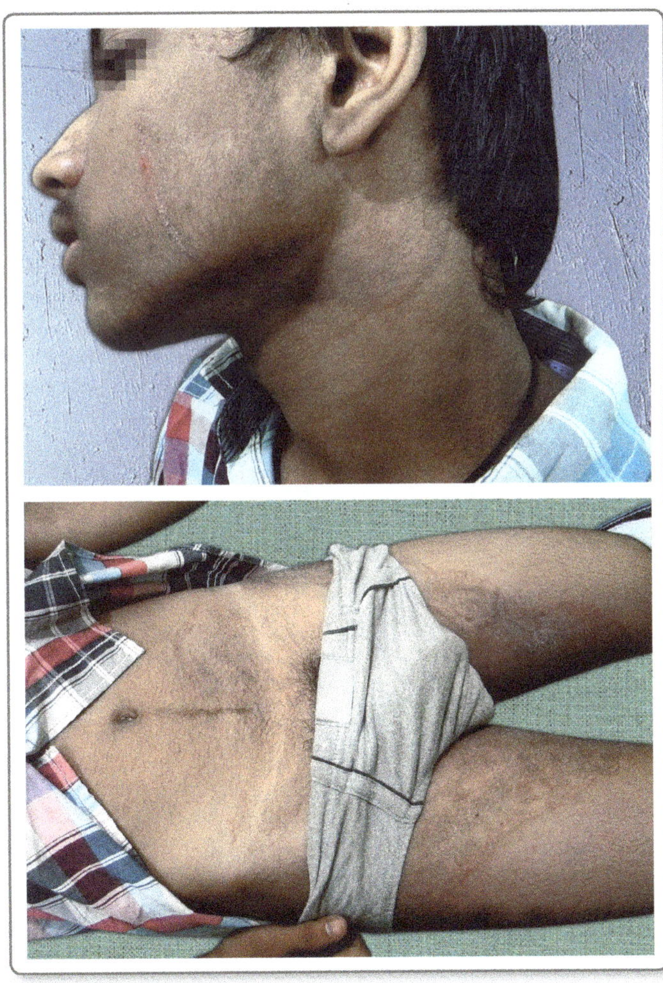

Q. What is the (i) diagnosis and (ii) management?

Answers

i. Tinea facei and corporis and cruris.

ii. Management

- Oral terbinafine 250 mg OD for 14 days
  or oral fluconazole 150 mg once/week for 4 weeks
  or oral itraconazole 200 mg OD for 14 days
- Topical terbinafine, ketoconazole or clotrimazole daily for 4 weeks.

Case 10

A 52-year-old lady had chronic eczematous lesions with central ulceration on medial aspect of left ankle for last 4 years. She had associated varicosity of leg veins for last 10 years.

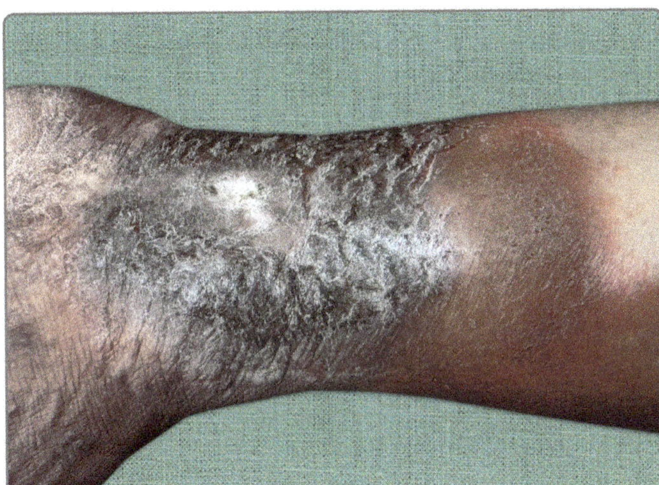

Q. What is the (i) diagnosis and (ii) management?

Answers

i. Stasis dermatitis with ulceration.

ii. Management

- Management of varicose veins by stockings, crepe bandage, etc.
- Avoidance of topical application (higher chance of contact sensitivity)
- Swab from the wound for bacterial culture and sensitivity
- Sterile normal saline cleansing
- Oral antibiotic when needed
- Oral antihistamines
- Topical emollient (without paraben, fragrance and lanolin) on eczematous area.

Case 11

A 19-year-man developed sudden onset vesicles ('dew-drop on rose petal' like) followed by pustules and crusting on face and upper part of trunk and limb with oral enanthem and history of preceding phase of fever and malaise.

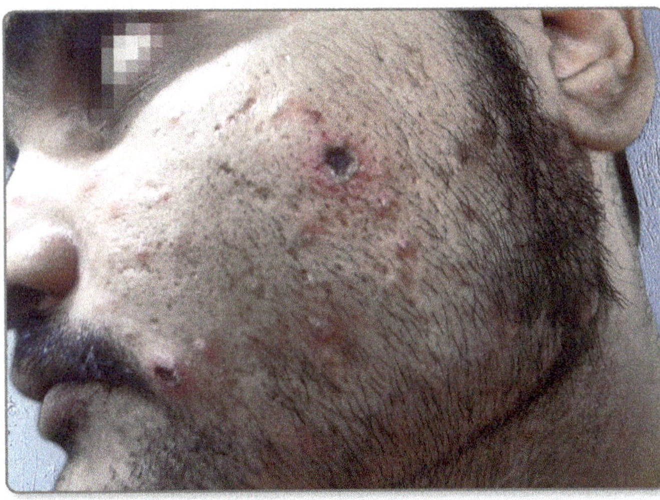

Q. What is the (i) diagnosis and (ii) management?

Answers

i. Varicella (Chickenpox).

ii. Management

- Adult varicella is to be always be treated by oral antivirals to prevent secondary complications (especially viral pneumonia)
- Oral valacyclovir 1000 mg thrice daily for 7 days or acyclovir 800 mg 5 times a day for 7 days or famciclovir 500 mg 8 hourly for 7 days
- Oral antibiotics preferably macrolides for 5–7 days to prevent secondary infection.

Case 12

A 29-year-old male had multiple verrucous lesions on beard area for last 3 months which are spreading fast. He had history of saloon-shaving before the episode.

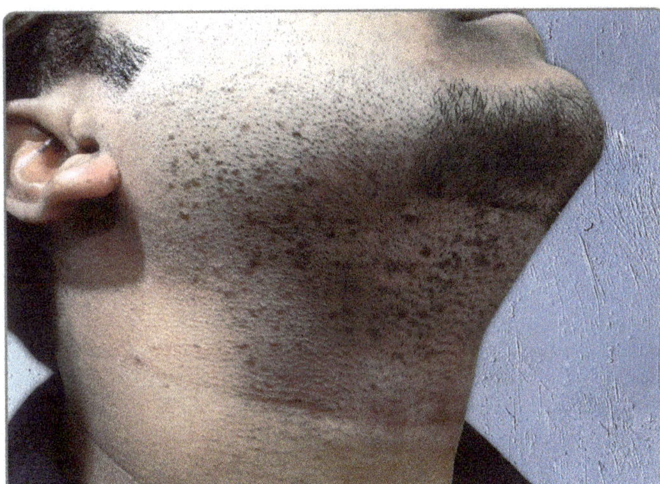

Q. What is the (i) diagnosis and (ii) management?

Answers

i. Verruca plana.

ii. Management

- Tretinoin 0.05% (keratolytic) to be applied by tooth-pick at evening for 2–3 hours daily
- If delayed response chemical cautery (by 80% tricloroacetic acid) or light electrocautery by experienced dermatologist.

Case 13

A 32-year-old man had skin rash on waist line and lower abdomen for last 3 months. He had history of application of topical corticosteroids for last 2 months. The lesions were subsided apparently at the beginning but spreaded on the periphery and ultimately did not heal. On examination, mild scaly lesions without any active inflammatory border along with some depigmented patches (arrow) were seen.

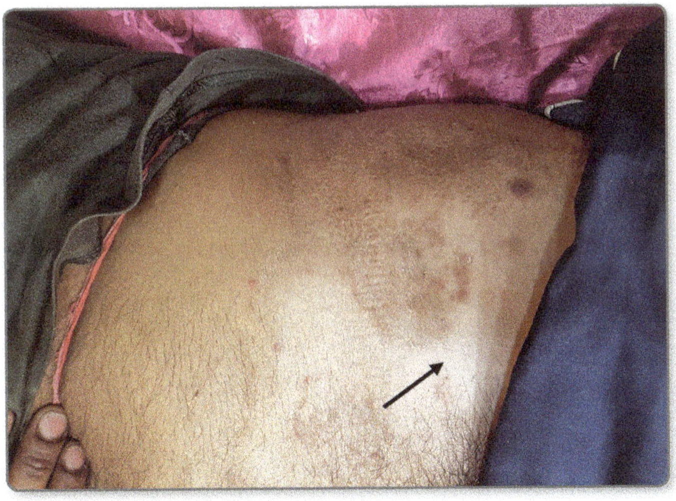

Q. What is the (i) diagnosis and (ii) management?

Answers

i. Tinea incognito or steroid-modified tinea (topical corticosteroid suppressed the inflammatory border and thus, the typical annular border and central clearing of tinea lesions were masked here. Topical corticosteroids caused the depigmentation).

ii. Management

- Strict avoidance of topical corticosteroids
- Oral terbinafine 250 OD for 15 days
  or, oral fluconazole 150 mg once/week for 4 weeks
  or, oral itraconazole 100 mg BD for 14 days
- Topical terbinafine, amorolfine, sertaconazole, or luliconazole daily for 4 weeks.

Case 14

A 53-year-old female had acneiform lesions with open comedones on face especially around eyes and temple for last 1 year.

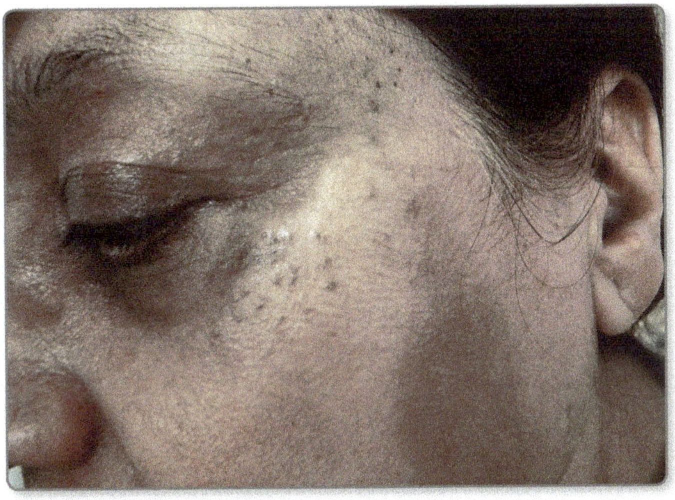

Q. What is the (i) diagnosis and (ii) management?

Answers

i. Senile acne.

ii. Management

- Tretinoin 0.05% (keratolytic) to be applied by tooth-pick at evening for 2–3 hours daily
- If delayed response removal of comedones by comedo-extractor.

Case 15

A 24-year-old female had terminal hairs on chin area for last 3 years. She had history of irregular menstruation for last 5 years.

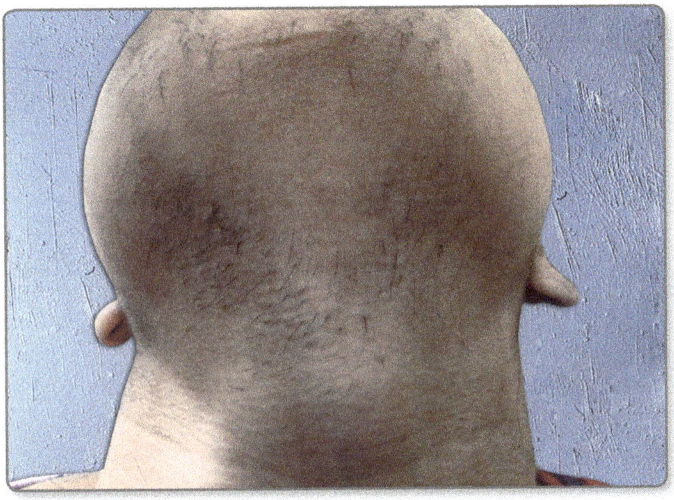

Q. What is the (i) diagnosis and (ii) management?

Answers

i. Hirsutism.

ii. Management

- Referral to gynecologist/endocrinologist to exclude polycystic ovarian diseases (PCOD), etc. as underlying cause
- Eflornithine hydrochloride cream twice daily for 3–6 months under monitoring on affected skin
- Lasor or electro-epilation by experienced dermatologist.

Case 16

A 21-year-old young male had erythematous scaly lesions with crusting bilaterally on face for last 1 year. He had no oral lesions.

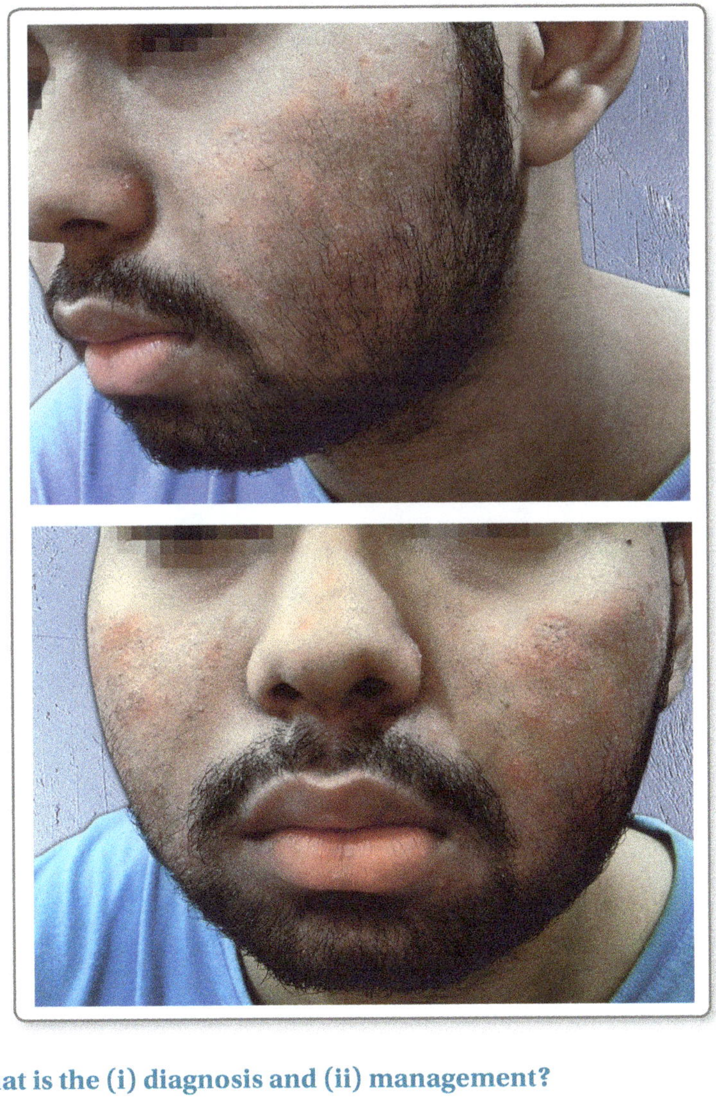

Q. What is the (i) diagnosis and (ii) management?

Answers

i. Pemphigus erythematosus.
ii. Management
- Referral to dermatologist
- Skin biopsy to confirm diagnosis
- To exclude associated LE (by ANA test)
- Topical potent steroid
- High dose of corticosteroids with adjuvant immunosuppressant under experienced dermatologist care.

Case 17

A 63-year-old female had acute erythematous eruption on face, forearms and V-area of neck aggravated by sun exposure, reddish patch around eyelids ('heliotrop erythema') for last 6 months alongwith proximal myopathy for last 1 month. She had also eryhematous papules on knuckles of hands ('Gottron's papules').

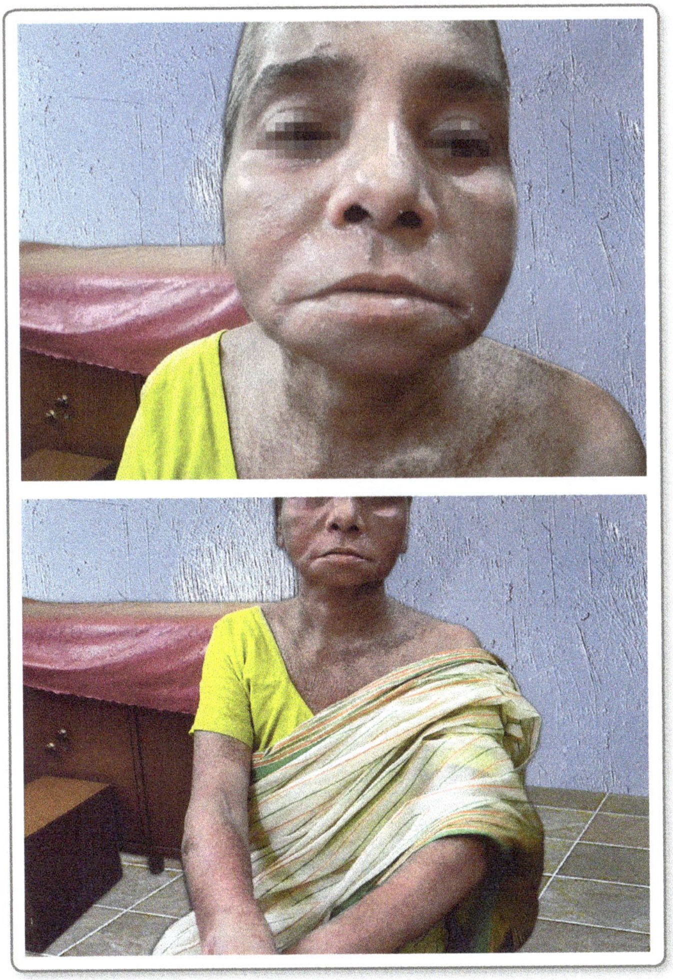

Q. What is the (i) diagnosis and (ii) management?

Answers

i. Dermatomyositis.
ii. Management
   - Referral to dermatologist and rheumatologist
   - Skin biopsy and muscle biopsy to confirm diagnosis
   - To exclude associated SLE
   - High dose of corticosteroids with adjuvant immunosuppressant under experienced dermatologist and rheumatologist care.

Case 18

A 27-year-old male had sudden onset pruritic erythematous eczematous lesions on both underarms sparing the vault of the axillae (black arrow) for last 1 week . He had history of wearing a new shirt for last 2 weeks.

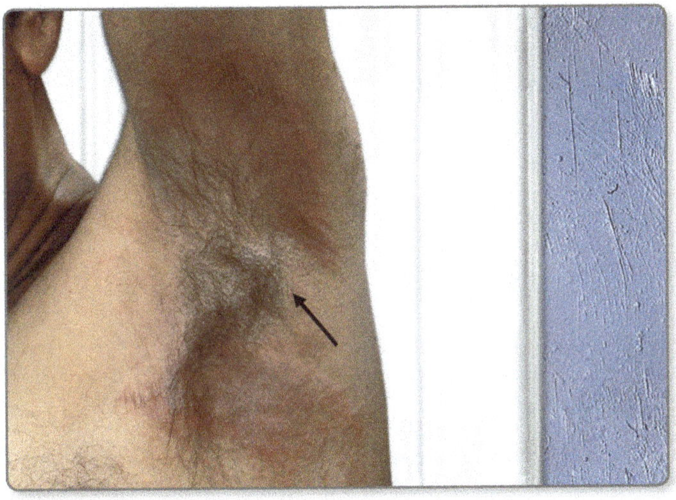

Q. What is the (i) diagnosis and (ii) management?

Answers

i. Allergic contact dermatitis (ACD) from the textiles (in ACD from deodorants vault of the axillae are affected).

ii. Management
- Strict avoidance of the offending shirt
- Mid-potent topical corticosteroids twice daily for 14 days
- Oral antihistamines for 7 days.

Case 19

A 21-year-old male had hypertrophic lesions on shoulder for 6 months. He had also acneiform eruption on face and trunk or last 4 years.

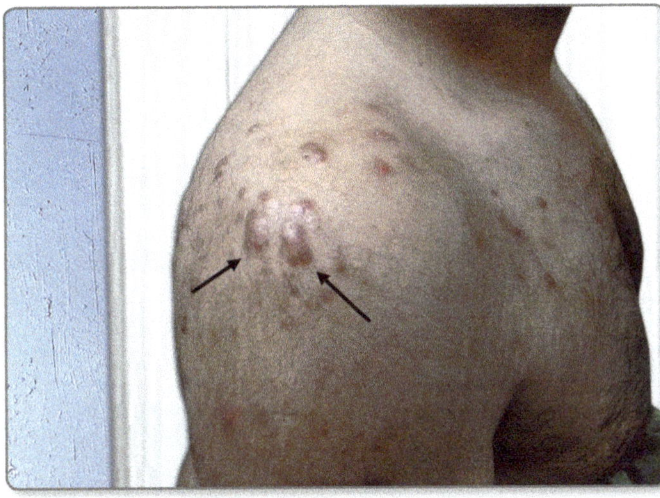

Q. What is the (i) diagnosis and (ii) management?

Answers

i. Acne keloidalis.

ii. Management

- Treatment of acne: Oral isotretinoin, topical benzoyl peroxide
- Intralesional corticosteroid by expert dermatologist with or without silicon gel sheet application.

Case 20

A 59-year-old male had sudden onset painful and tender erythematous plaque on left side of face alonwith similar two lesions on trunk for last three months. The trunkal lesions were hypoesthetic. He had faint hypopigmented patches on same sites for last about 2 years.

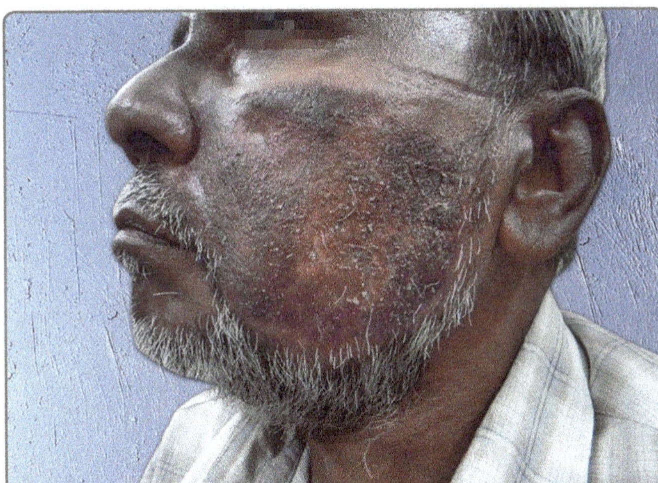

Q. What is the (i) diagnosis and (ii) management?

Answers

i. Leprosy: Borderline tuberculoid (BT) with type I reaction.
ii. Management
- Multidrug treatment (MDT) consisting of dapsone 100 mg daily, clofazimine 50 mg daily, rifampicin 600 mg monthly (supervised)
- Oral prednisolone 60 mg OD to be tapered over 6 to 8 weeks.

Case 21

A 21-year-old obese male had non-pruritic, vevety thickened skin on neck for last 3 years. He had strong family history of diabetes in both his parents.

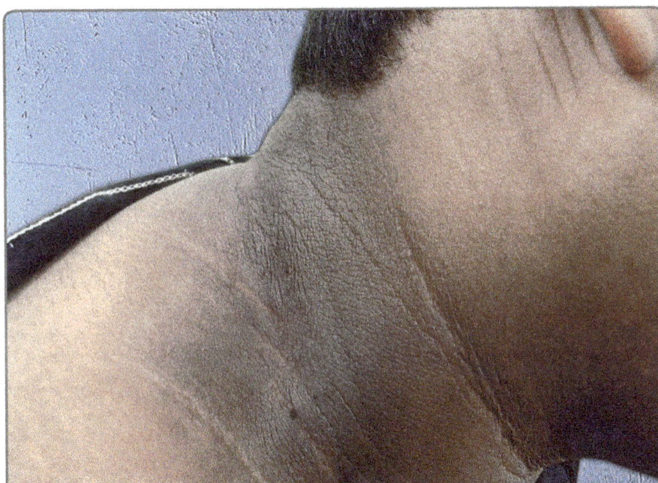

Q. What is the (i) diagnosis and (ii) management?

Answers

i. Acanthosis nigricans.

ii. Management
- To measure serum insulin level, blood sugar profile
- Reduce obesity
- Regular physical exercise
- Oral metformin if serum insulin level is high
- Topical tretinoin 0.5% cream on affected area once at night gently.

Case 22

A 35-year-old male palmoplantar well-defined scaly plaques (yellow arrow) for last 2 years aggravating in winter with nail pittings. He has also dactylitis (red arrow) and terminal interphalangeal joint involvement and deformity (white arrows).

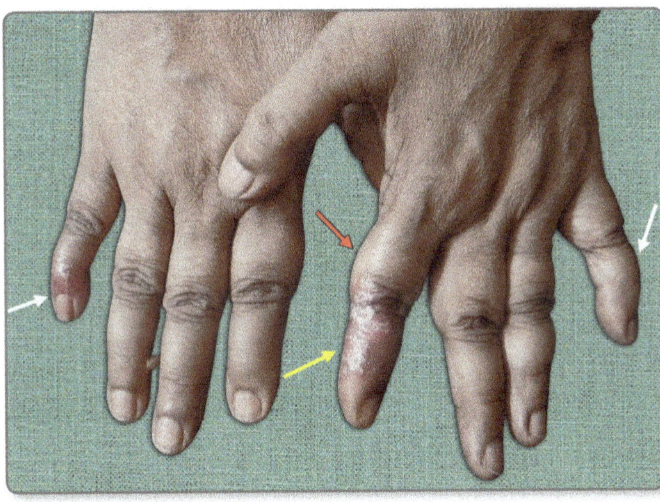

Q. What is the (i) diagnosis and (ii) management?

Answers

i. Psoriasis with psoriatic arthritis (PsA).
ii. Management
   - Referral to dermatologist and rheumatologist
   - Oral methotrexate under their supervision
   - Topical potent steroid followed by topical calcipotreine locally on skin plaques once daily
   - Topical emollients locally once daily.

Case 23

A 41-year-old man, diabetic, had pruritic scaly eruption on both feet especially involving interdigital areas for last 2 years which used to be aggravated during summer and rainy season.

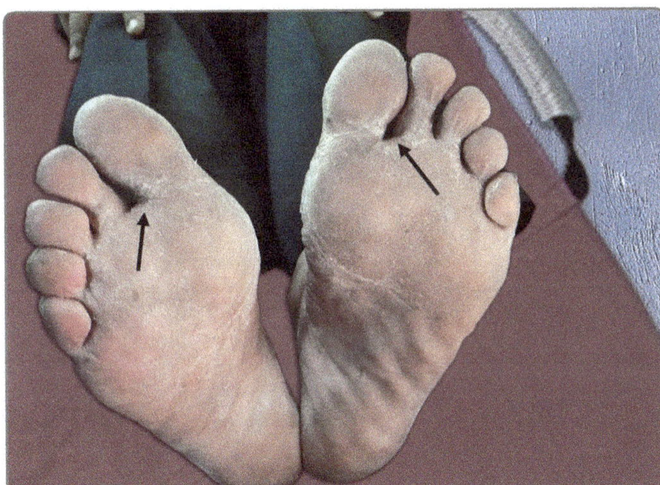

Q. What is the (i) diagnosis and (ii) management?

Answers

i. Tinea pedis.

ii. Management

- Oral terbinafine 250 mg OD for 14 days
  or oral fluconazole 150 mg once/week for 4 weeks
  or oral itraconazole 200 mg OD for 14 days
- Topical terbinafine, ketoconazole or clotrimazole daily for 4 weeks
- To keep the feet dry
- To use cotton socks and airy loose-fitting shoes.

Case 24

A 31-year-old man had history chronic erosive papulovesicular lesions on groins and axillae for last 20 years mostly aggravating during summar and rainy season. He had strong family history of similar diseases in his family. Topical and systemic antifungal treatment did not help him at all.

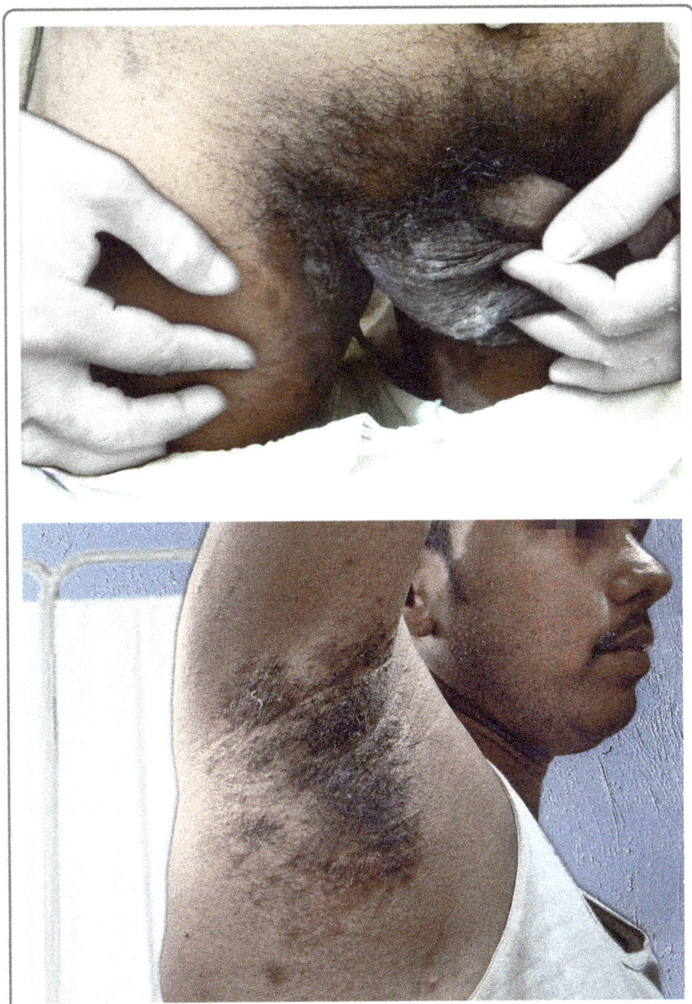

Q. What is the (i) diagnosis and (ii) management?

Answers

i. Hailey-Hailey disease.

ii. Management

- Minimizing friction and sweating
- Emollient containing antibacterials
- Soap substitutes
- Antiseptic bath additives
- Moderately potent topical corticosterois with or without antibacterials and antifungals.

Case 25

A 54-year-old male had chronic pruritic erythematous lichenified (thickening of the skin, increased criss-cross markings of skin looking like 'lichen') lesions on both lower legs and dorsum of feet for last 3 years.

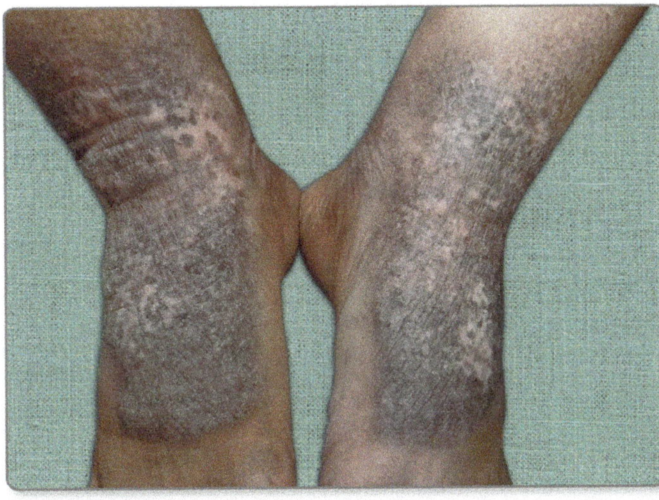

Q. What is the (i) diagnosis and (ii) management?

Answers

i. Lichen simplex chronicus.

ii. Management

- Topical superpotent topical corticosteroids for 2 weeks followed by low potent corticosteroids for 6 weeks
- Oral antihistamines (preferably sedative antihistamines).

Case 26

A 14-year-old male had generalized dry 'fish-like' scales sparing flexors (black arrow) since infancy which used to aggravate in winter. He had history of similar illness in his father.

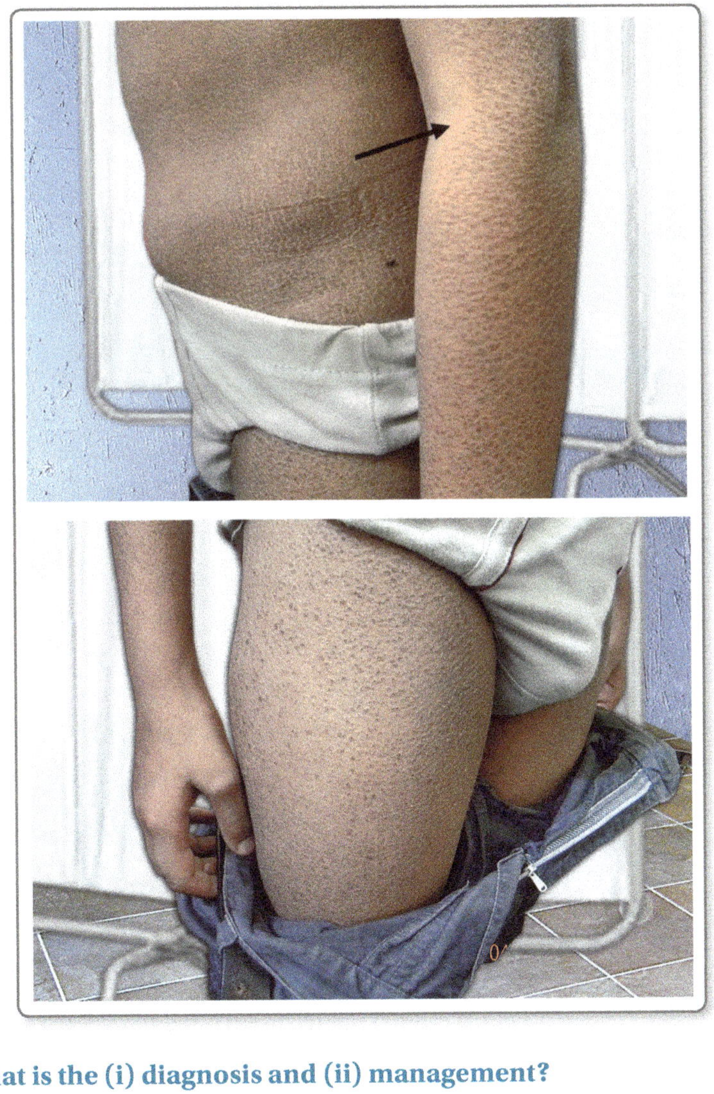

Q. What is the (i) diagnosis and (ii) management?

Answers

i. Ichthyosis vulgaris.

ii. Management

- Skin hydration by adequate bath followed by immediate application of moisturizer
- Mild keratolytics like salicylic acid, lactic acid, urea and propylene glycol application.

Case 27

A 31-year-old man had pruritic purpuric eruption for last 4 days. The purpura were palpable. He had history of taking a NSAID (nimesulide) 1 week back for joint pain.

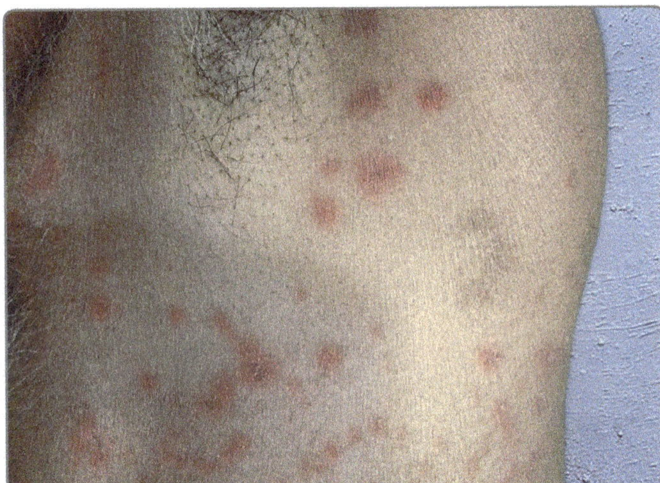

Q. What is the (i) diagnosis and (ii) management?

Answers

i. Allergic purpura.

ii. Management
  - Withdrawal of the offending drug
  - Strict avoidance of the offending drug
  - Urine screening for RBC to exclude renal involvement
  - Exclusion of systemic involvement
  - Oral antihistamines
  - Topical calamine lotion
  - Topical mid-potent corticosteroid
  - If refractory: Oral corticosteroids (short course).

Case 28

A 28-year-old lady had diffuse scarring alopecia for last 6 months. On examination minute keratotic papules were seen at the hair foliicles.

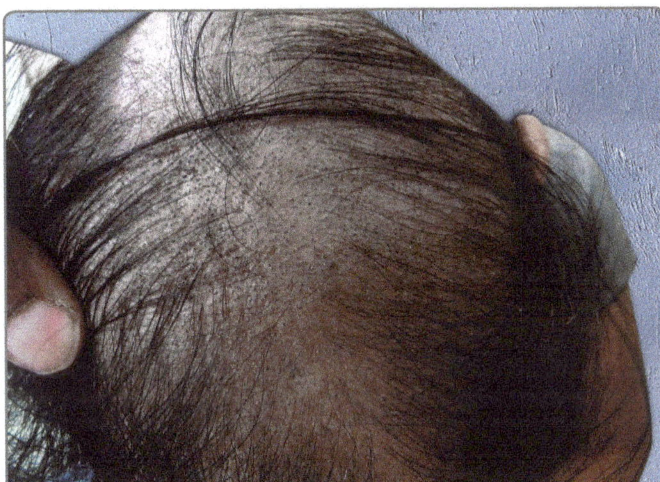

Q. What is the (i) diagnosis and (ii) management?

Answers

i. Lichen planopilaris.

ii. Management
- Referral to dermatologist
- Histopathological confirmation of diagnosis
- High potent topical corticosteroids
- Systemic corticosteroids (30–40 mg) for 12 weeks.

Case 29

A 54-year-old male had pruritic multiple papular eruption with central keratotic plug (white arrows) predominantly on extensor surface of the limbs for last 3 months. He had been suffering from uncontrolled diabetes.

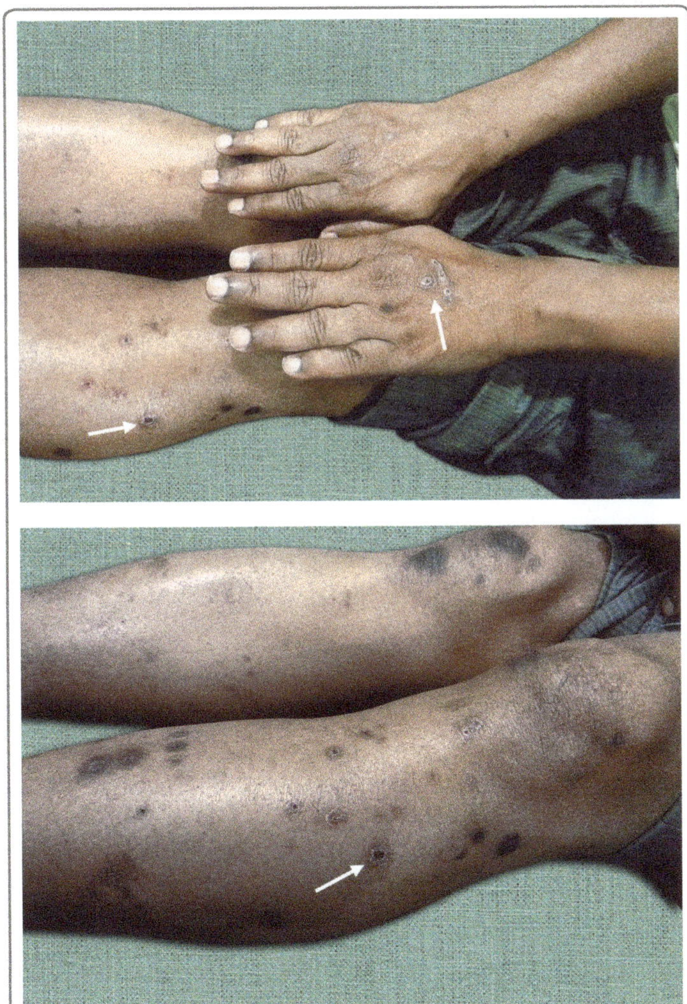

Q. What is the (i) diagnosis and (ii) management?

Answers

i. Perforating folliculitis.

ii. Management

- Referral to endocrinologists to control diabetes
- Topical tretinoin 0.025% (gradually increased to 0.05%) to apply at evening
- PUVA by expert dermatologist.

Case 30

A 49-year-old female had an asymptomatic localized hyperpigmented plaque on front of the right side of the chest. On examination sclerosis was found in the whole lesion.

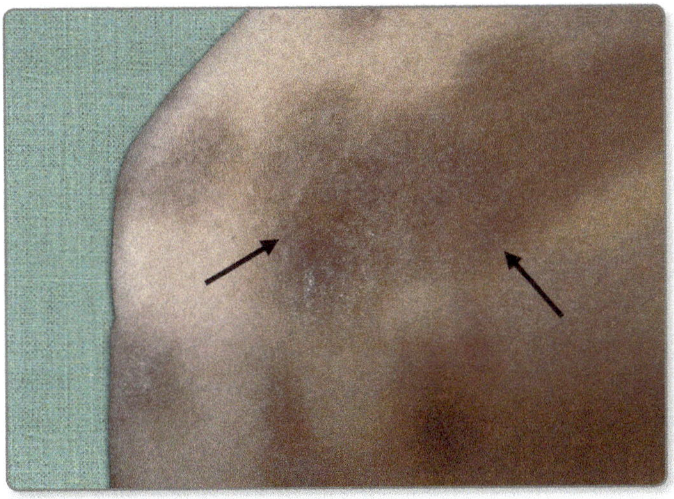

Q. What is the (i) diagnosis and (ii) management?

Answers

i. Morphea (localized scleroderma).

ii. Management
   - Referral to dermatologist
   - Topical or intralesional corticosteroids
   - Topical calcipotriol.

Case 31

A 58-year-old male had sudden development of asymptomatic depigmented lesions on forehead and other part of face for last 6 weeks. On examination some confetti macules (black arrows) were seen adjacent to the lesions. He had history of application of hair dye containing para-phenylenediamine (PPD) for last 6 months.

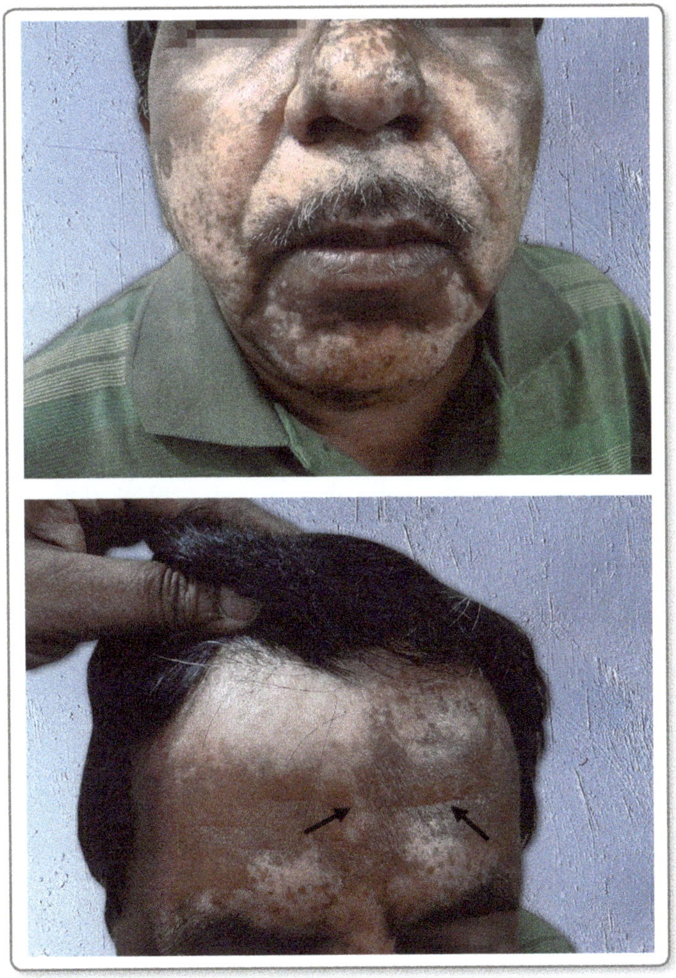

Q. What is the (i) diagnosis and (ii) management?

Answers

i. Chemical leukoderma.

ii. Management

- Strict avoidance of dye containing PPD
- Topical mid-potent steroid once daily or topical tacrolimus 0.1% or topical pimecrolimus twice daily
- If refractory UVB narrow band or PUVA or PUVAsol under expert dermatologist.

Case 32

A 29-year-old female had multiple, discrete, tiny, glistening, flesh-colored smooth and flat, round papules on arms and neck for last 3 months.

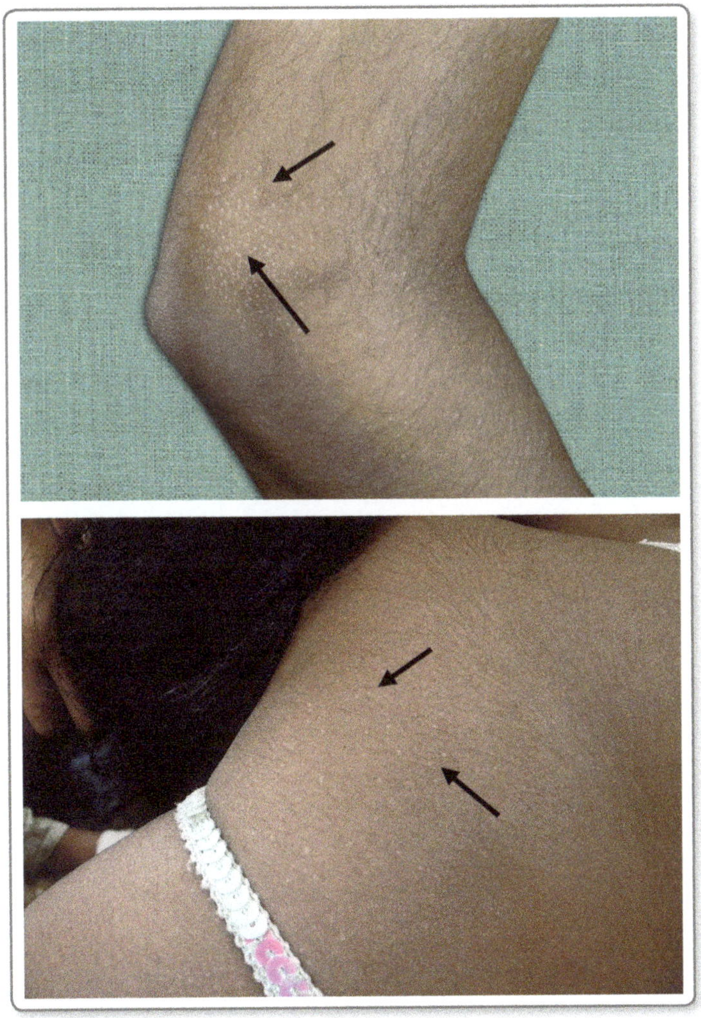

Q. What is the (i) diagnosis and (ii) management?

Answers

i. Lichen nitidus.

ii. Management

- Topical mid-potent corticosteroid
- Oral antihistamines (if pruritus).

Case 33

A 24-year-old young lady had a linear hyperpigmented asymptomatic mark in geometric shape on dorsum of left hand for about last 10 days. Her parents gave the history of her marriage negotiation which she did not approve. On repeated investigations she confessed that she has produced the lesion by application of bathroom-cleansing acid.

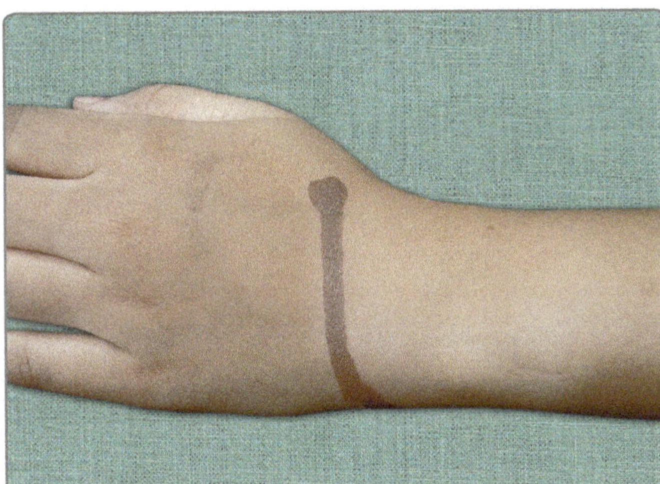

Q. What is the (i) diagnosis and (ii) management?

Answers

i. Dermatitis artefacta.

ii. Management

- A supportive, nonconfrontational, empathic approach
- Referral to psychiatrist
- Mid-potent topical corticosteroid once daily
- Day-time sunscreen.

Case 34

A 31-year-old lady had persistent facial erythema, flushing alongwith papules and pustules predominantly on convex area for last 3 years.

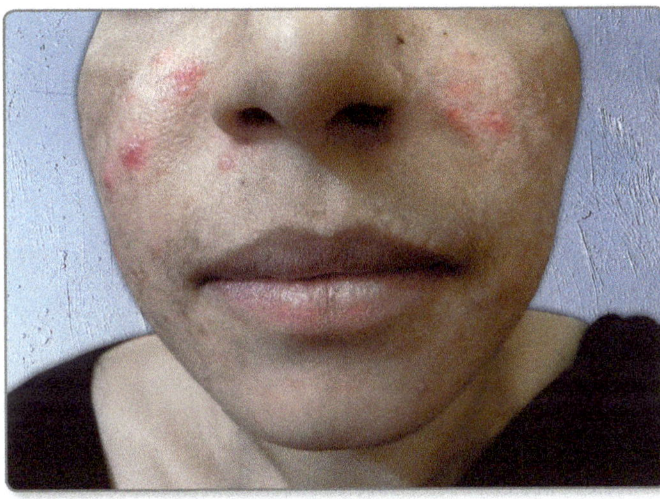

Q. What is the (i) diagnosis and (ii) management?

Answers

i. Rosacea.

ii. Management

- Topical metronidazole 1% gel twice daily or azelaic acid 15% once daily
- Topical benzoyl peroxide gel or wash, clindamycin gel or pimecrolimus cream or tacrolimus ointment
- Oral doxycycline (low dose: 40 mg daily) or tetracycline (low dose: 250 mg BD) or isotretinoin (low dose: 10–40 mg daily)
- Oral macrolides or metronidazole.

Case 35

A 19-year-old young man had asymptomatic linear atrophic lesion on left axilla for last 3 months. He had history of application of topical steroid and antifungal combination for last 6 months intermittently for itching and rash on axillae.

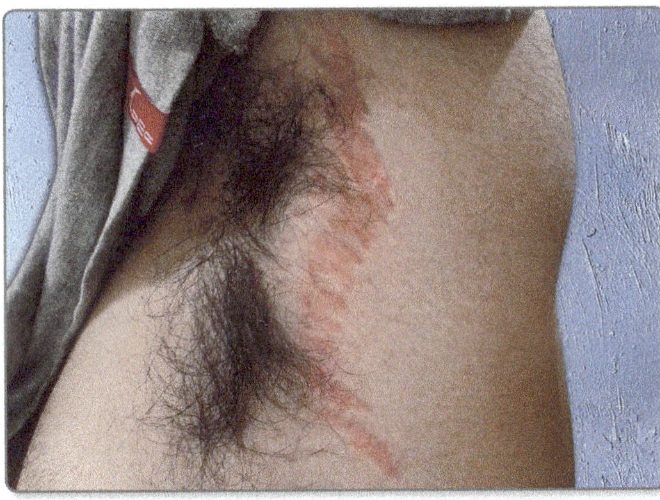

Q. What is the (i) diagnosis and (ii) management?

Answers

i. Striae (steroid-induced).

ii. Management

- Strictly avoidance of topical steroid preparation
- Topical tretinoin 0.025% (gradually increased to 0.05%) daily in evening gently.

Case 36

A 27-year-old lady had thick, hyperkeratotic lesions on feet for last one year. On examination the lesions were more tender on lateral pressure than ventral pressure.

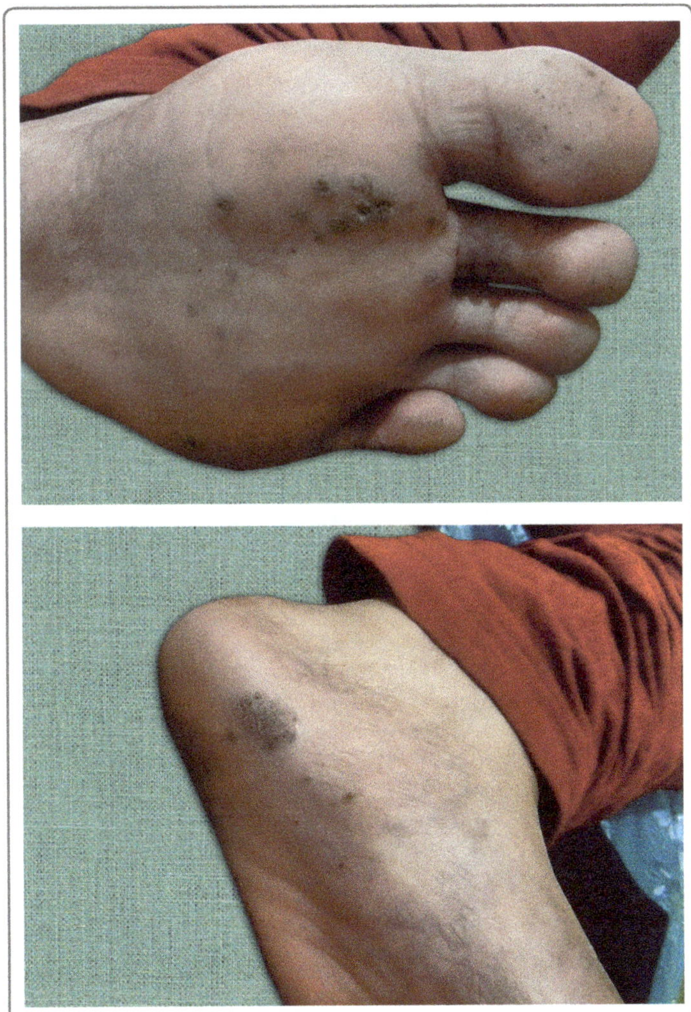

Q. What is the (i) diagnosis and (ii) management?

Answers

i. Plantar verruca.

ii. Management

- Salicylic acid 16.5%
  Lactic acid 16.5%
  Flexible collodion 10 mL
  Mft pig.
  To apply on the warts with applicator for 2–3 hours (later overnight)
- Topical antibacterial once a day
- If refractory, chemical cautery (by 80% trichloroacetic acid), electrocautery or cryosurgery by trained dermatologist.

Case 37

A 36-year-old lady had gradually developing alopecia in parting region for last 1 year. Her frontal and temporal hair margins are well preserved.

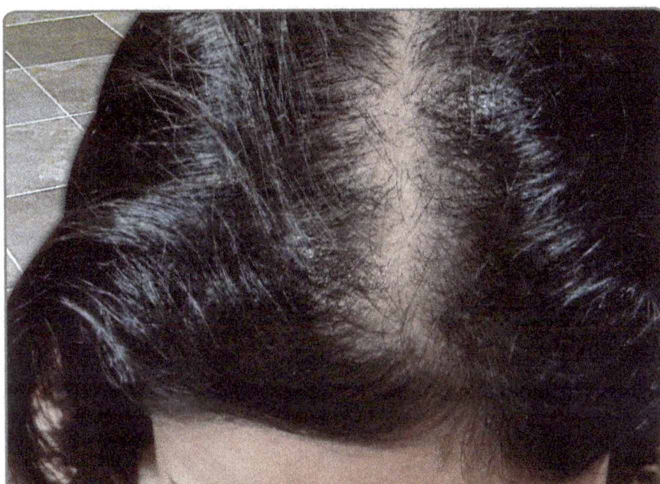

Q. What is the (i) diagnosis and (ii) management?

Answers

i. Female pattern hair loss (Olssen type).
ii. Management
   - Screening for hematological, gynecological and endocrinological status
   - Topical minoxidil 2% lotion 1 mL twice daily for 6 months.

Case 38

A 57-year-old man had gradually developing alopecia predominantly involving temporal area for last 5 years.

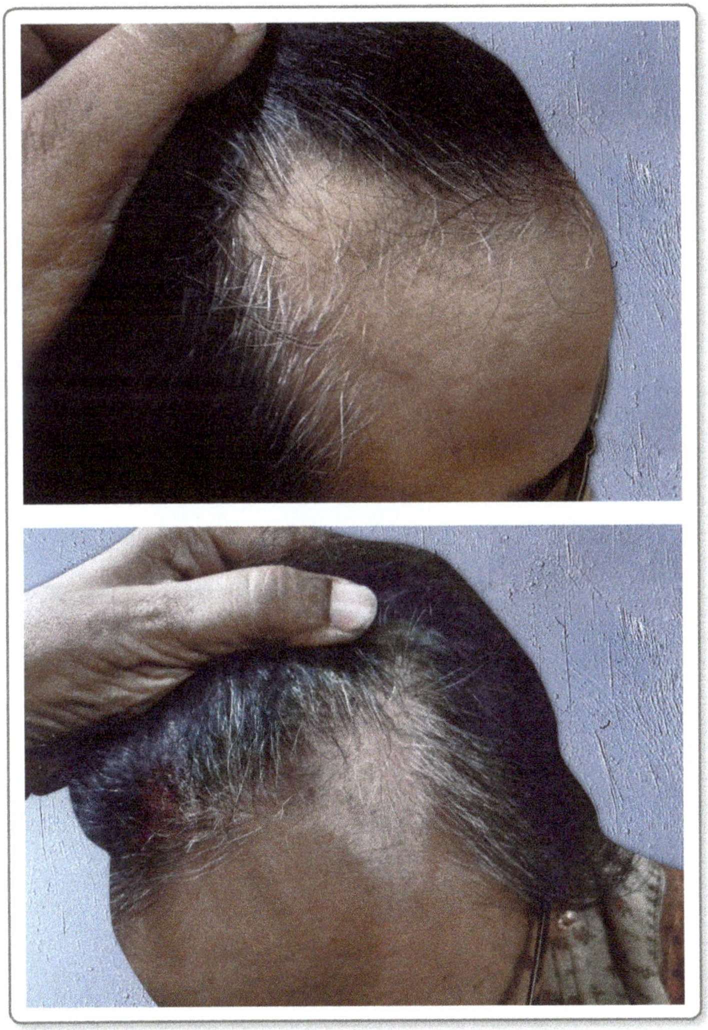

Q. What is the (i) diagnosis and (ii) management?

Answers

i. Male pattern hair loss (MPHL) or AGA (Hamilton-Norwood type).

ii. Management

- Topical minoxidil 5% lotion 1 mL twice daily for 6 months
- Oral finasteride 1 mg daily under supervision of expert dermatologist.

Case 39

A 39-year-old lady had itchy unilateral lesion on left side of face with active inflammatory border (arrow) and central clearing for last 6 weeks.

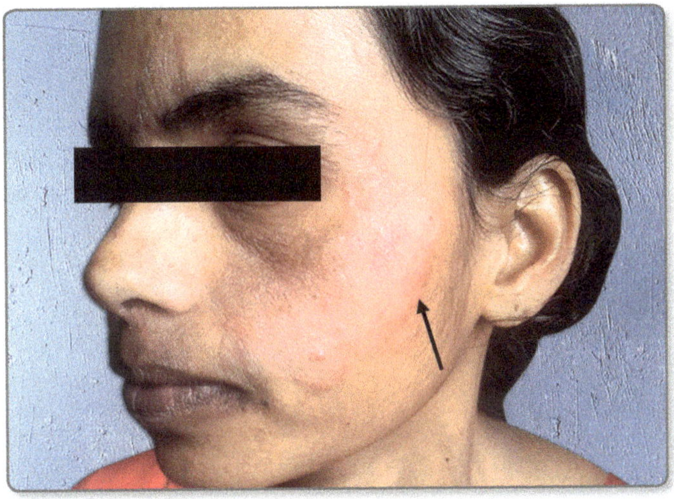

Q. What is the (i) diagnosis and (ii) management?

Answers

i. Tinea faciei.

ii. Management

- Oral terbinafine 250 OD for 15 days
  or, oral fluconazole 150 mg once/week for 4 weeks
  or, oral itraconazole 100 mg BD for 14 days
- Topical terbinafine, sertaconazole, luliconazole, or amorolfine daily for 4 weeks.

Case 40

A 27-year-old male had severe inflammatory papulopustules and nodules on face with massive scarring and hyperpigmentation for last 8 years.

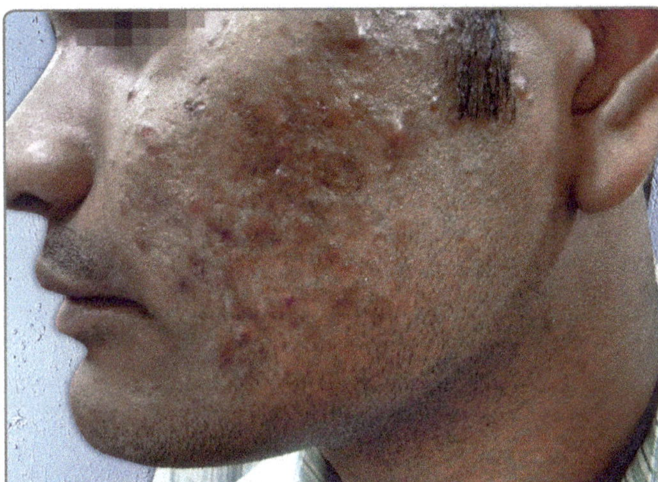

Q. What is the (i) diagnosis and (ii) management?

Answers

i. Acne nodularis.

ii. Management

- Oral isotretinoin 20 mg twice daily by pre-therapy screening and per-therapy monitoring for lipid and liver enzymes level for 3 to 6 months
- Topical clindamycin twice daily for 2 months
- Topical benzoyl peroxide 2.5% gel daily once daily for 6 months
- After completion of acne treatment scar management.

Case 41

A 25-year-old male had extensive acneiform eruption (black arrows) on arms, back and chest for last 1 year. The lesions had no comedone and he had no acneiform lesions on face. He had history of application of topical steroid on and off during last 3 years.

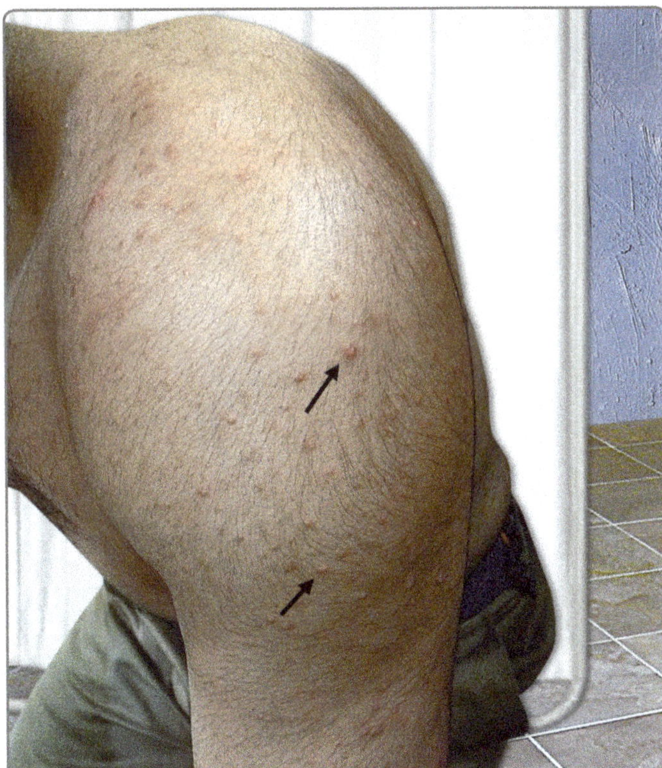

Q. What is the (i) diagnosis and (ii) management?

Answers

i. Steroid acne or folliculitis.

ii. Management
  - Strict avoidance of topical steroid
  - Topical benzoyl peroxide 2.5% gel to apply at evening daily for 3 months
  - Oral doxycycline, if refractory.

Case 42

A 41-year-old female had itchy, scaly lesion with annular shape and active inflammatory border (arrow) on dorsum of right hand with involvement of interdigital folds for last 2 months.

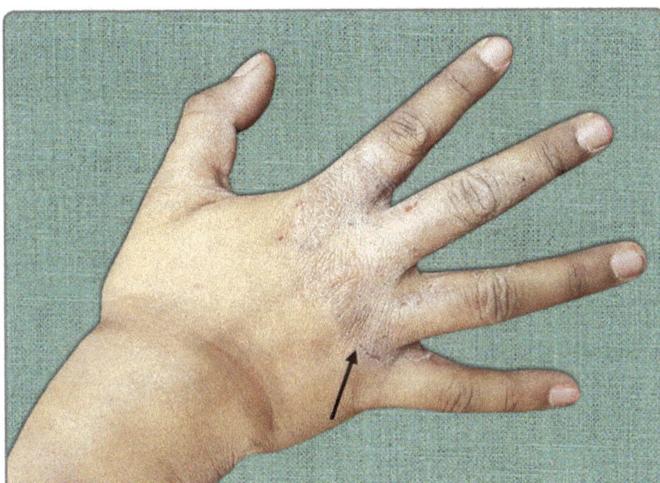

Q. What is the (i) diagnosis and (ii) management?

Answers

i. Tinea manuum.

ii. Management

- Oral terbinafine 250 OD for 15 days
  or oral fluconazole 150 mg once/week for 4 weeks
  or oral itraconazole 100 mg BD for 14 days
- Topical terbinafine, sertaconazole, luliconazole or amorolfine daily for 4 weeks.

Case 43

A 41-year-old male had history bluish appearance of toes and fingers on exposure of cold for last 10 years and tightening (sclerosis) (black arrow) of facial and acral skin for last 3 years. The tip of her digits had become narrow (white arrows).

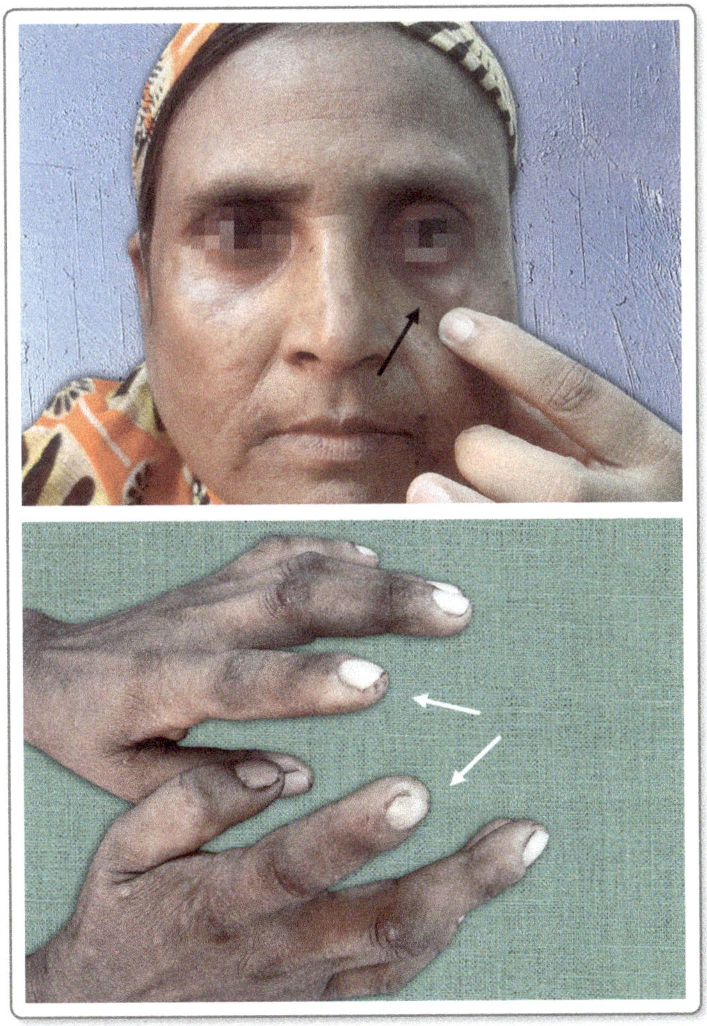

Q. What is the (i) diagnosis and (ii) management?

Answers

i. Systemic scleroderma (limited) [lcSsc].
ii. Management
- Referral to dermatologist and rheumatologist
- Avoidance of cold exposure (to use woolen gloves, socks, etc.)
- To monitor systemic involvement especially renal and pulmonary organs.

Case 44

A 9-year-old girl had small superficial vesicles (white arrow) on face for last 10 days. The vesicles ruptured to form superficial erosions with yellowish-brown crust (black arrow).

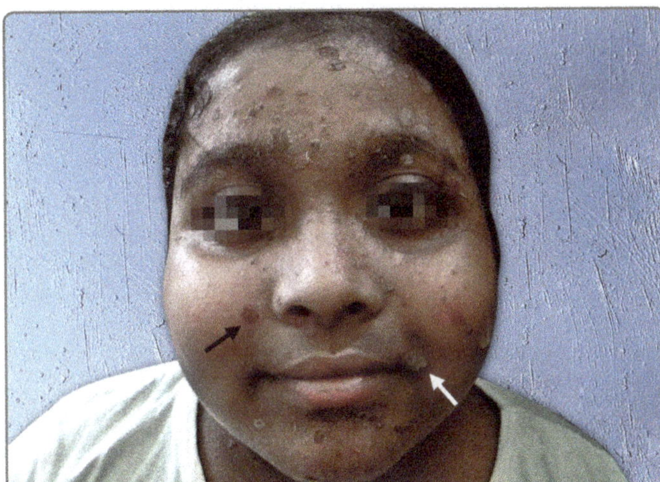

Q. What is the (i) diagnosis and (ii) management?

Answers

i. Impetigo vulgaris.

ii. Management

- Topical retapamulin or mupirocin or fusidic acid
- Oral cloxacillin, cephalexin, or erythromycin
- To watch for nephropathy in later weeks (beta-hemolytic *Streptococcus*, frequent cause of impetigo, may induce glomerulonephritis in certain cases).

Case 45

A 32-year-old male had dark colored papules (white arrows) on his scrotum for last 10 years with history of occassional hemorrhage (seen on his undercloths as blood-stain). He had similar problem in his father.

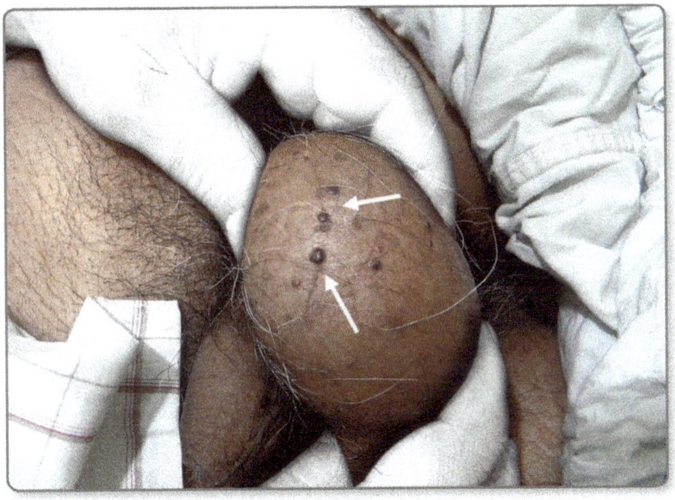

Q. What is the (i) diagnosis and (ii) management?

Answers

i. Angiokeratoma scroti.

ii. Management

- Referral to dermatologist
- Light electrofulguration or cryotherapy.

Case 46

A 34-year-old male had acute pruritic erythematous wheals (black arrow) on face and different parts of the body and limbs for last 3 days. He had no history of associated breathing difficulty and choking throat. He had taken food in a restaurent 4 days back.

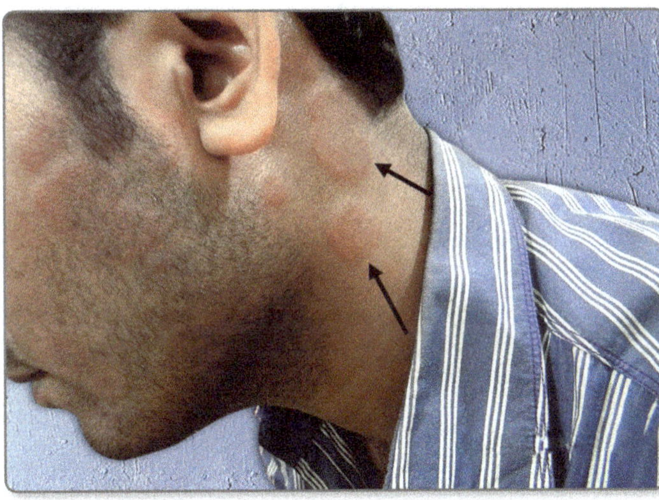

Q. What is the (i) diagnosis and (ii) management?

Answers

i. Acute urticaria (probably due to food-additives).
ii. Management
   - Strict avoidance of outside food and NSAIDs
   - To watch for acute respiratory symptoms (then immediate emergency hospitalization)
   - Oral antihistamines (if not responding dose escalation)
   - Short course of systemic steroid, if refractory.

Case 47

A 53-year-old male had recurrent oral (black arrow) and genital ulceration for last 5 years. Pathergy test by intradermal normal saline produced positive result (white arrow).

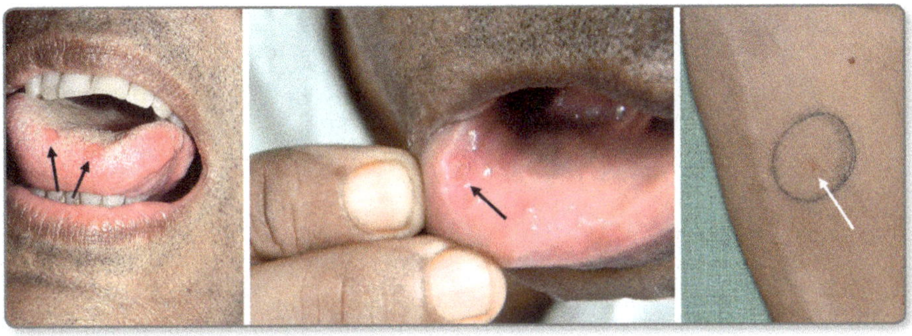

Q. What is the (i) diagnosis and (ii) management?

Answers

i. Behcet's disease.
ii. Management
   - Referral to dermatologist and rheumatologist (to exclude systemic organ involvement especially large vessels and CNS)
   - Topical chlorhexidine mouthwash, topical corticosteroids, topical sucralfate
   - Oral tetracycline suspension
   - Oral colchicin or dapsone (under experienced dermatologist).

Case 48

A 45-year-old male, farmer by profession, had pruritic papulovesicular eruption on face, trunk and limbs for last 2 years mostly aggravated during rainy season. His submental area (white arrow) were spared. He had history of exposure to parthenium plants during his occupation.

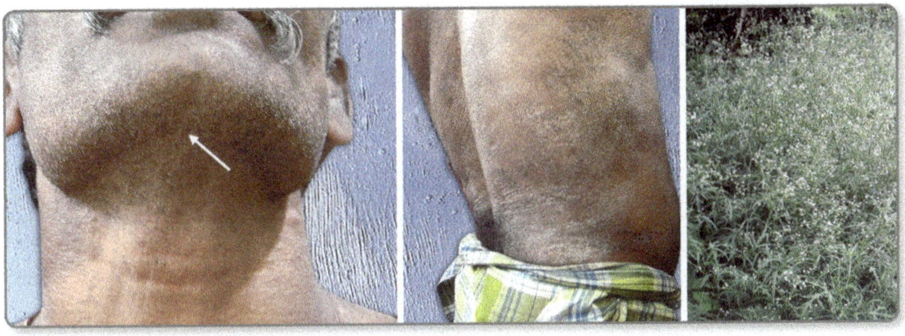

Q. What is the (i) diagnosis and (ii) management?

Answers

i. Photoallergic contact dermatitis (PACD) to parthenium (in airborne contact dermatitis or ABCD submental and retroauricular area are spared).

ii. Management
   - To avoid parthenium and sun exposure as far as possible by using full sleeves, etc.
   - Topical low potent steroid or tacrolimus on face
   - Topical potent steroid on trunk and limbs
   - Antihistamines
   - Oral short course steroid, if refractory.

Case 49

A 54-year-old female had pruritic violaceous flat-topped papules (white arrows) on thighs, legs, dorsum of feet for last 1 year. On examination her buccal mucosa showed lacy pattern of whitish plaque (black arrow).

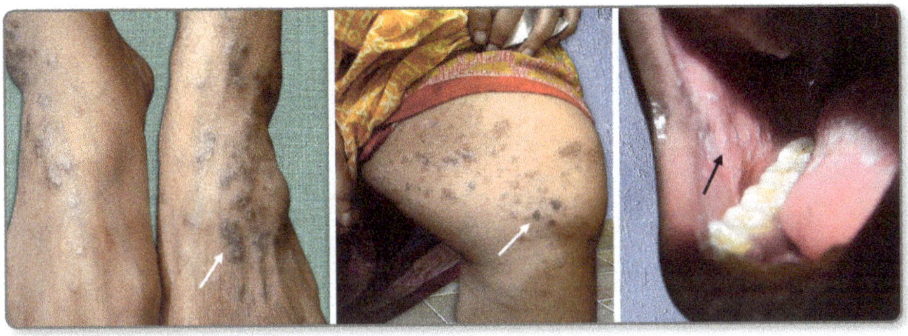

Q. What is the (i) diagnosis and (ii) management?

Answers

i. Lichen planus.

ii. Management

- To avoid oral dental metal fitting, amalgam, if any
- Topical potent steroid on trunk and limbs
- Antihistamines
- Oral short course steroid, if refractory.

Case 50

A 43-year-old female had nodular swelling on lower leg (posterior) for last 2 years. Her Mantoux test (5 TU) produced strong positive (18+) result

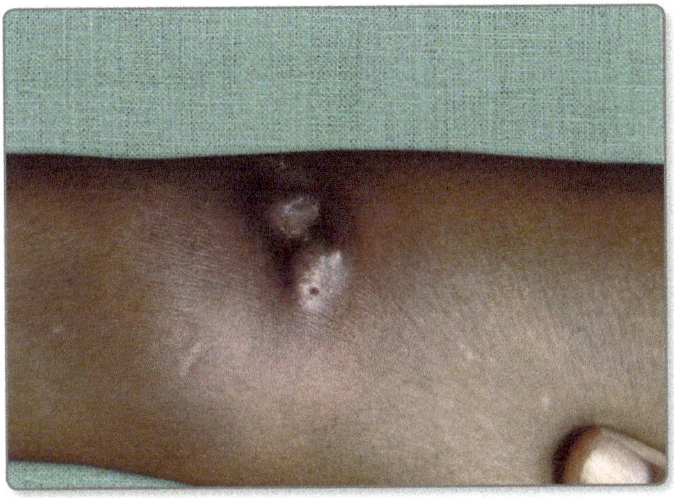

Q. What is the (i) diagnosis and (ii) management?

Answers

i. Erythema induratum of Bazin (if PCR from tissue biopsy shows evidence of *Mycobacteria tuberculosis*) or nodular vasculitis (if PCR of *Mycobacteria tuberculosis negative*).

ii. Management
   - Referral to experienced dermatologist
   - Management depends on histopathology and PCR report.

Case 51

A 37-year-old lady had frontal alopecia in temporal area with receding hair margin and also severe acne and scar on face for last 6 years. She had also polycystic ovarian disease (PCOD) for last 10 years.

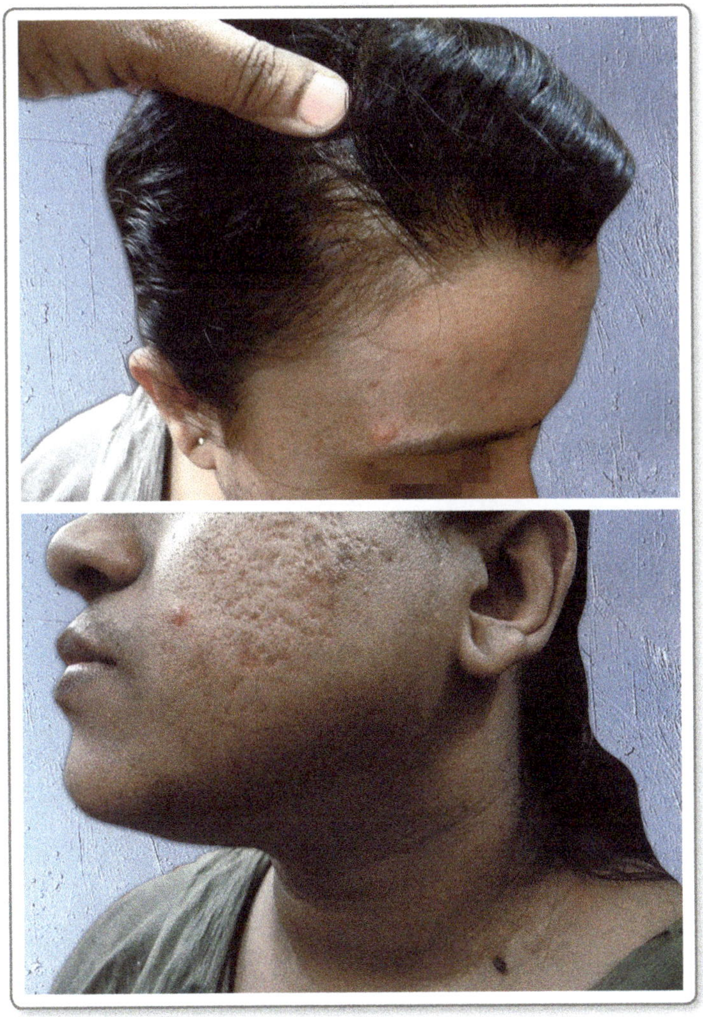

Q. What is the (i) diagnosis and (ii) management?

Answers

i. Male pattern hair loss (Hamilton-Norwood type) and adult acne due to PCOD.

ii. Management
   - Management of PCOD by gynecologist/endrocrinologist
   - Minoxidil 2% lotion 1 mL twice daily on scalp for 6 months
   - Oral doxycycline 100 mg OD or minocycline 100 mg OD for 2–3 months
   - Topical benzoyl peroxide, clindamycin and tretinoin/adaferin on face
   - Acne scar management.

Case 52

A 35-year-old lady had extensive hyperpigmented, lichenoid eruptions on limbs for last 5 years. On examination there were linear arrangement of pigmented papules (white arrows) within the lesion.

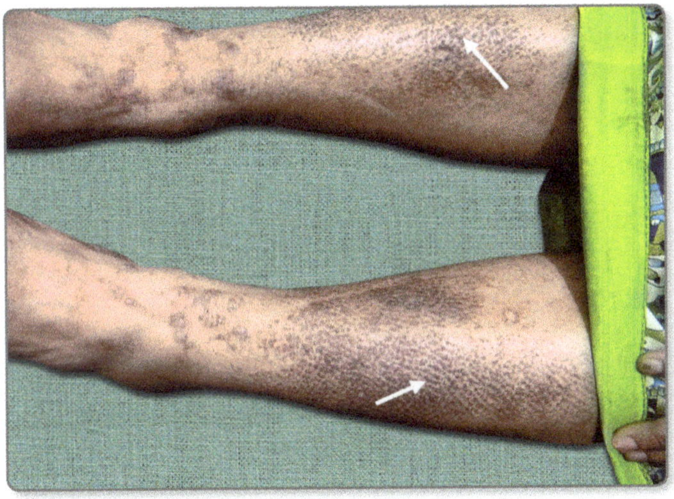

Q. What is the (i) diagnosis and (ii) management?

Answers

i. Lichen amyloid.

ii. Management

- Avoidance of 'bath-scrubbers' on skin
- Topical potent steroid with or without salicylic acid.

Case 53

A 32-year-old male had recurrent boils on different parts of skin for last 3 months. He has no history of diabetes mellitus or any immunosuppressing diseases or drug exposure.

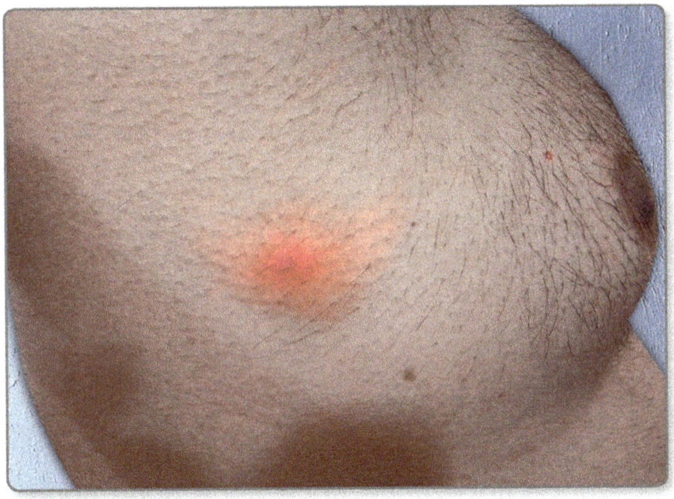

Q. What is the (i) diagnosis and (ii) management?

Answers

i. Recurrent furunculosis.

ii. Management

- Oral linezolid 600 mg twice daily for 7 days
- Topical retapamulin twice daily for 7 days
- Topical mupirocin cream once daily on carrier sites (anterior nares, external auditory meatus, axillae, umbilicus, groin and inner-buttock cleft) for 7 days/every month for 3 months
- If refractory oral rifampicin 450 to 600 mg orally with amoxicillin 500 mg thrice daily for 10 to 14 days.

Case 54

A 68-year-old lady had been suffering from recurrent oral ulcer for last 1 year followed by generalized flaccid blister with erosions for last 4 months. On examination Nikolsky's sign (lateral pressure on skin causes epidermal detachment) was positive (black arrow).

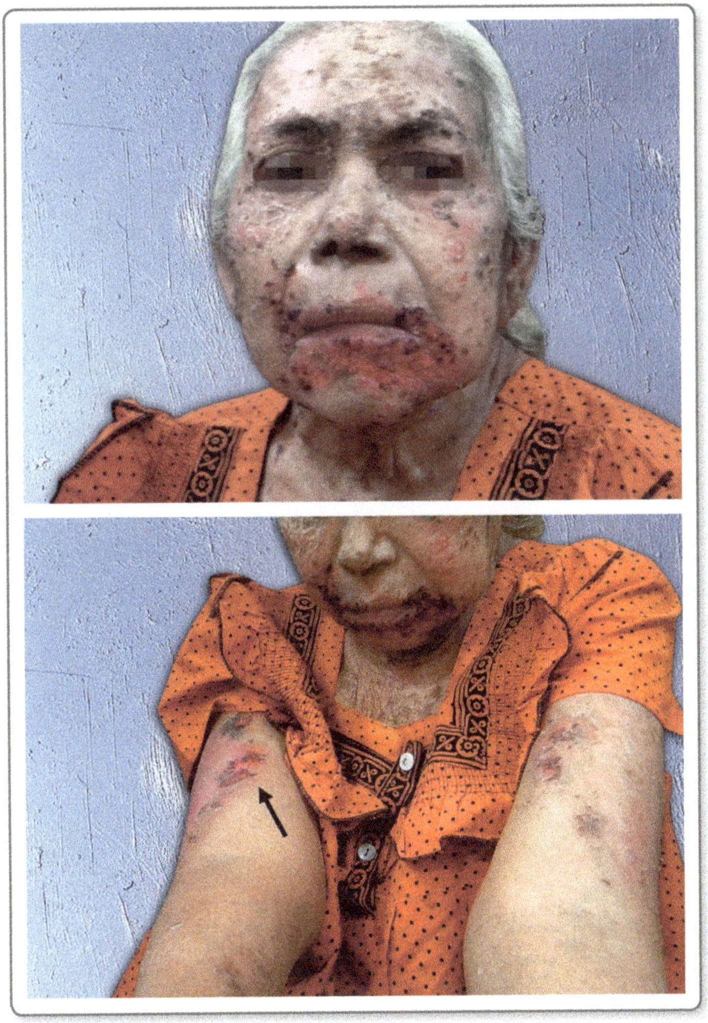

Q. What is the (i) diagnosis and (ii) management?

Answers

i. Pemphigus vulgaris.

ii. Management

- Referral to expert dermatologist
- Hospitalization
- Skin biopsy to confirm the diagnosis
- High dose of systemic corticosteroids with adjuvants (azathioprin or mycophenolate mofetil) by strict monitoring

  or

- Dexamethasone-cycloposhamide (DCP) pulse therapy in center where facility available.

Case 55

A 32-year-old lady had recurrent painful acneiform eruption on her nape of the neck for last 6 months.

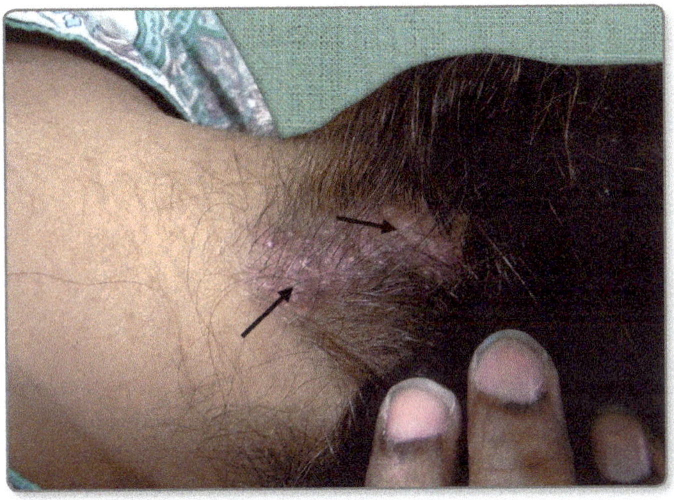

Q. What is the (i) diagnosis and (ii) management?

Answers

i. Acne keloidalis nuchae.
ii. Management
   - Oral doxycycline 100 mg or oral minocycline 100 mg daily for 2 to 3 months
   - Topical benzoyl peroxide or clindamycin gel.

Case 56

A lady had asymptomatic pigmented macules and patches for last 2 years on neck and upper trunk. Oral mucosa and nails were not affected.

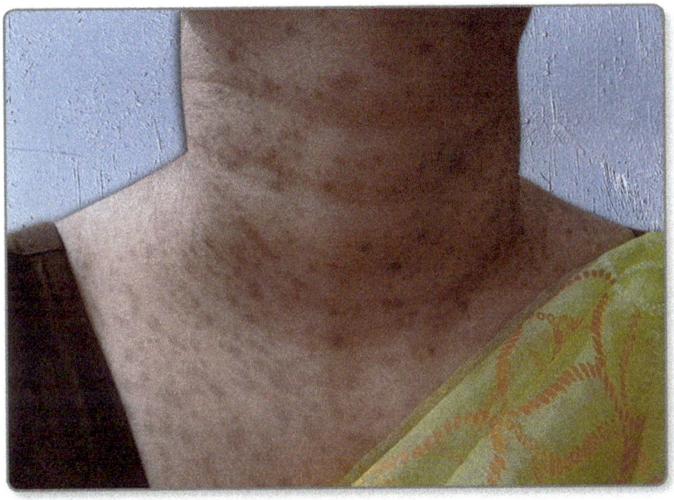

Q. What is the (i) diagnosis and (ii) management?

Answers

i. Lichen planus pigmentosus.
ii. Management
   - Broad spectrum sunscreen
   - Topical mid-potent corticosteroid.

Case 57

A 19-year-old girl had excessive sweating on hands and feet for last 5 years. She felt difficulty in writing and computer typing.

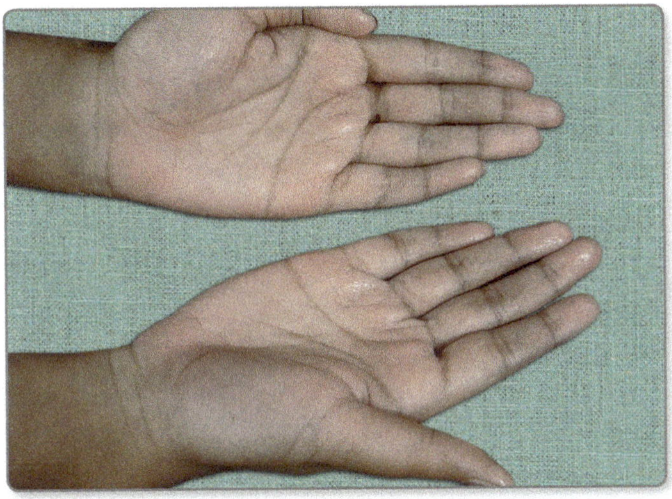

Q. What is the (i) diagnosis and (ii) management?

Answers

i. Palmoplantar hyperhidrosis.

ii. Management
  - Stress control
  - Topical aluminium chloride hexahydrate 20% in absolute alcohol to apply once at night
  - Tap water iontophoresis.

Case 58

A 51-year-old male asymptomatic, persistent, glistening moist shiny reddish patches on glans and inner prepuce (black arrows) for last 2 years.

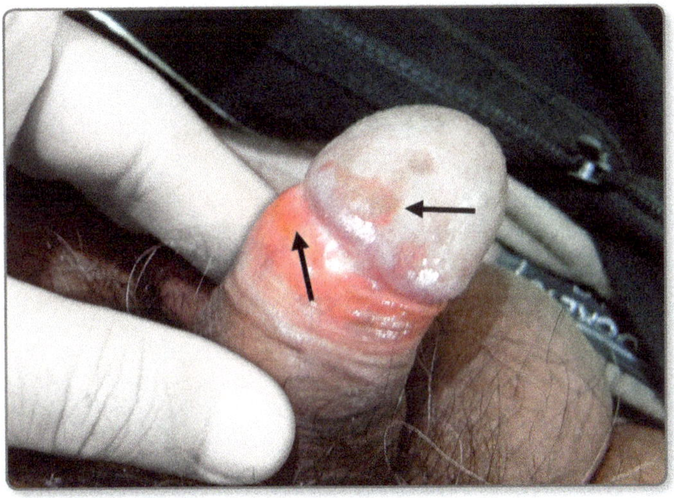

Q. What is the (i) diagnosis and (ii) management?

Answers

i. Zoon's (plasma cell) balanitis.

ii. Management
   - To improve washing habits and micturition practices
   - Intermittent application of mild to potent topical corticosteroids with or without antibacterials and antifungals
   - Topical tacrolimus
   - In refractory cases surgical circumcision.

Case 59

A 61-year-old male had recurrent painful pustular lesions on upper lip and beard for last 1 year. On examination perifollicular inflammation was seen.

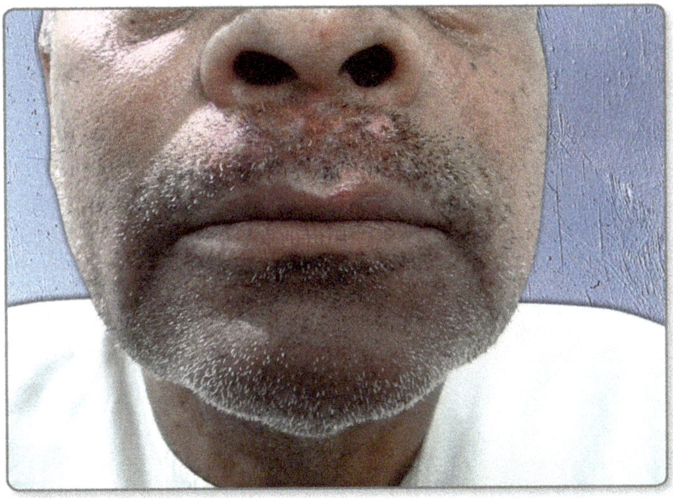

Q. What is the (i) diagnosis and (ii) management?

Answers

i. Sycosis barbae.
ii. Management
   - Warm saline compress
   - Avoid saloon shaving
   - Local antibiotic (retapamulin, mupirocin, or clindamycin)
   - Systemic antibiotic.

Case 60

A 28-year-old male had recurrent painful vesicular lesions followed by superficial erosions (black arrows) on glans for last 2 years. He had extra-marital partner.

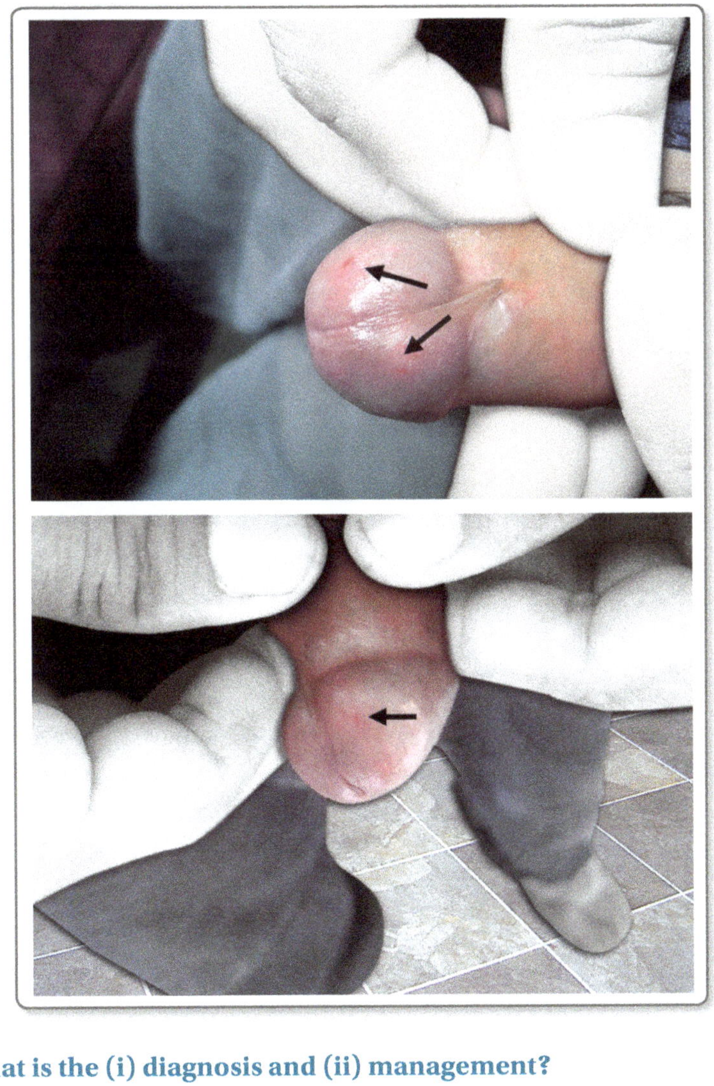

Q. What is the (i) diagnosis and (ii) management?

Answers

i. Recurrent herpes genitalis.

ii. Management

- To screen for other STDs especially HIV
- Supressive treatment (if recurrence 10 incidents/year):
  Oral valacyclovir 500 mg daily or 1,000 mg daily
  or oral acyclovir 400 mg twice daily
  or oral famcyclovir 250 mg twice daily
- Treatment duration: Upto 1 year.

Case 61

A 61-year-old male had tingling and numbness on anterolateral aspect of left thigh (on marked area) for last 6 months. On examination neither any skin patch nor any nerve thickening was detected.

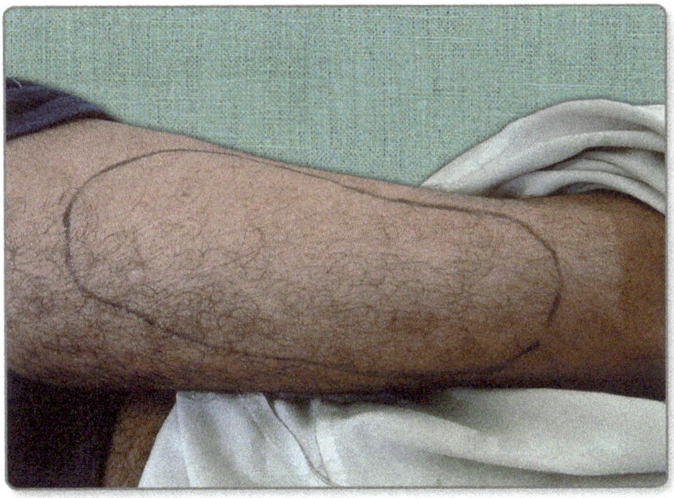

Q. What is the (i) diagnosis and (ii) management?

Answers

i. Meralgia paresthetica (Bernhardt's syndrome).

ii. Management

- Referral to orthopedic surgeon/neurologist.

Case 62

A 27-year-old male had asymptomatic progressively increasing generalized hypopigmented patches mostly on non-exposed skin for last 4 years.

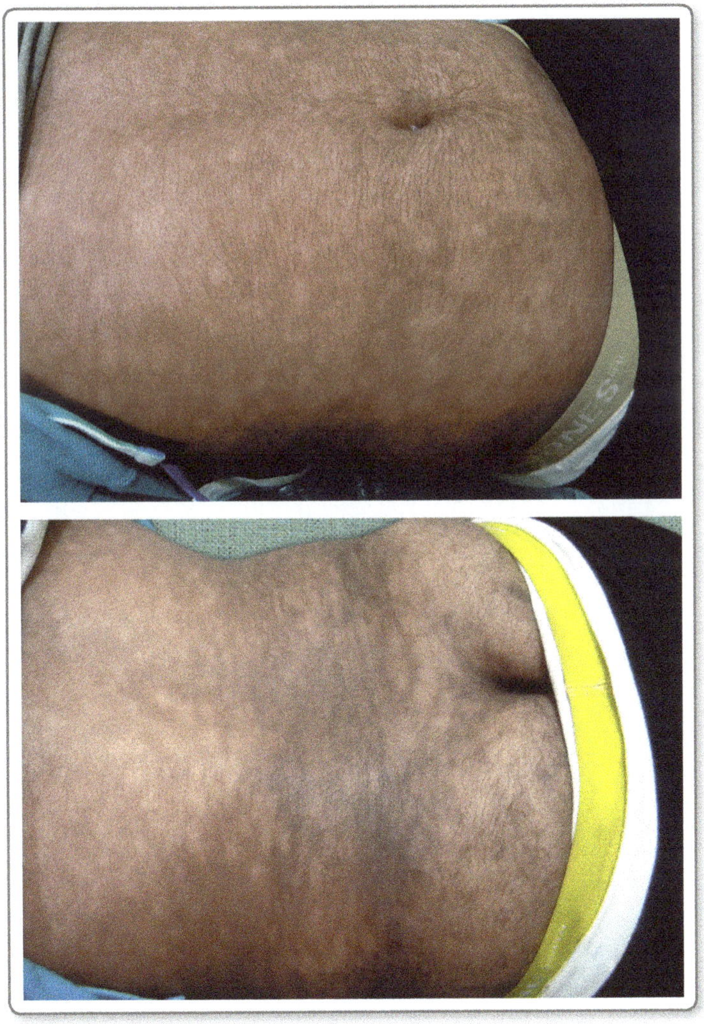

Q. What is the (i) diagnosis and (ii) management?

Answers

i. Mycosis fungoides (cutaneous T-cell lymphoma).

ii. Management
- Referral to experienced dermatologist
- To confirm diagnosis by histopathology and immunohistopathology
- Staging of the disease
- PUVA therapy or topical bexarotene or electron beam
- Systemic chemotharapy.

Case 63

A 27-year-old male had multiple pruritic, erythamatous papulovesicles (black arrows) on different parts of trunk and limbs for last 1 week. On examination the lesions had central puncta with surrounding areola (white arrow).

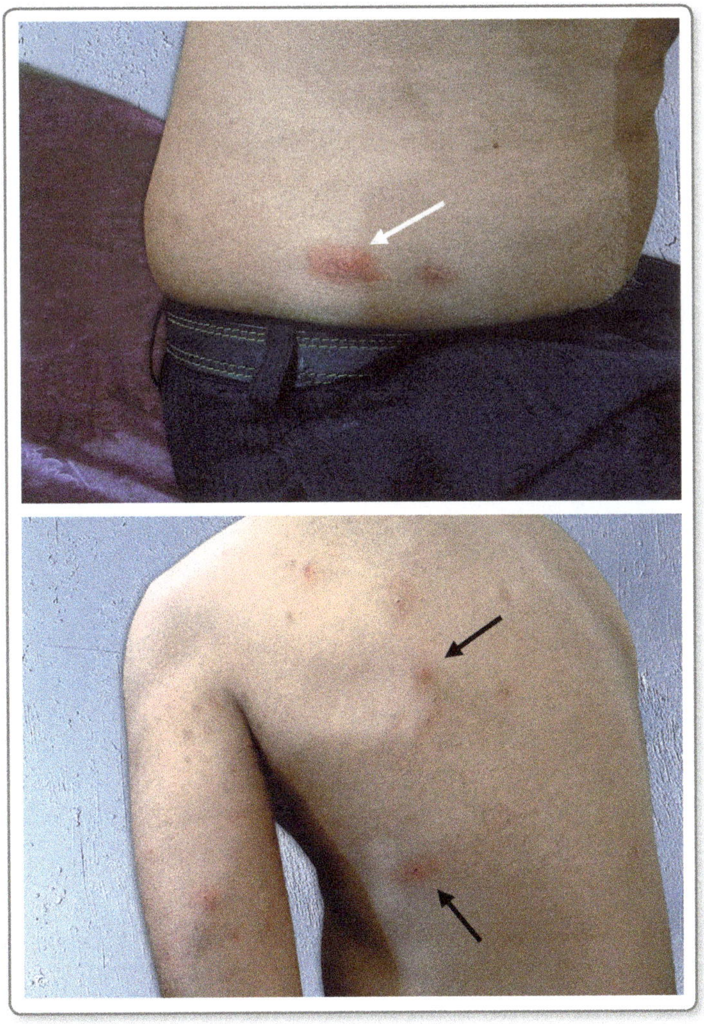

Q. What is the (i) diagnosis and (ii) management?

Answers

i. Insect allergy.

ii. Management

- To avoid insect exposure
- Topical mid-potent steroid with or without antibacterials
- Oral antihistamines.

Case 64

A 56-year-old lady had pruritic annular lesion on face for last 3 months. On examination the active border (black arrow) of the lesions showed papulovesicles and scales.

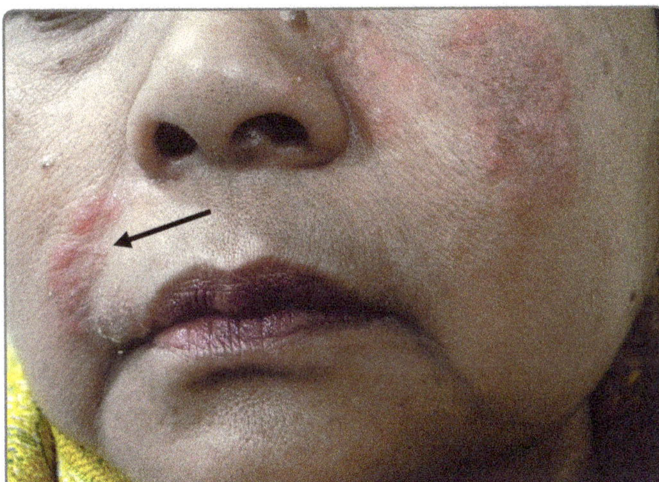

Q. What is the (i) diagnosis and (ii) management?

Answers

i. Tinea facei.

ii. Management

- Oral terbinafine 250 mg OD for 14 days
  or oral fluconazole 150 mg once/week for 4 weeks
  or oral itraconazole 200 mg OD for 14 days
- Topical terbinafine, ketoconazole, or clotrimazole daily for 4 weeks.

Case 65

A 17-year-old male had generalized asymptomatic nodules (black arrow), freckles (white arrows) and cafe-au-laits macules (blue arrow) on different parts of trunk and limbs.

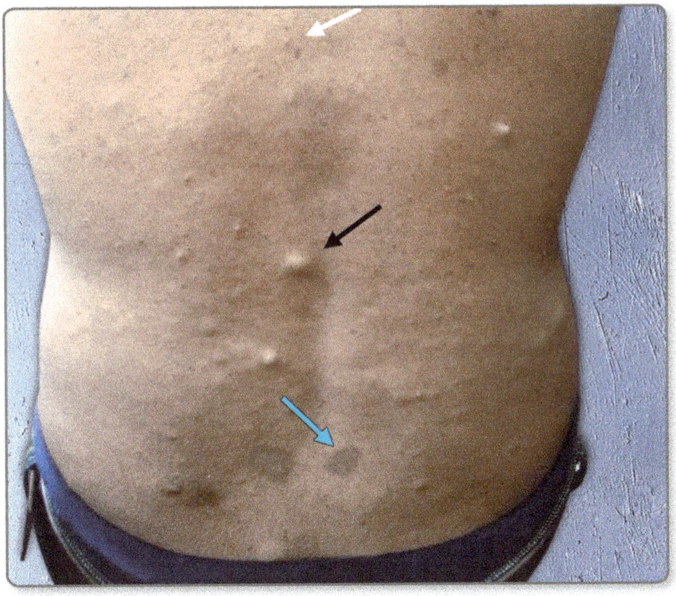

Q. What is the (i) diagnosis and (ii) management?

Answers

i. Neurofibromatosis.

ii. Management

- Counseling
- Referral to neurologist to exclude intracerebral involvement (CT Scan, MRI, etc.).

Case 66

A 32-year-old male had severe pruritus on scrotum for last 2 years. On examination the scotal skin showed lichenification.

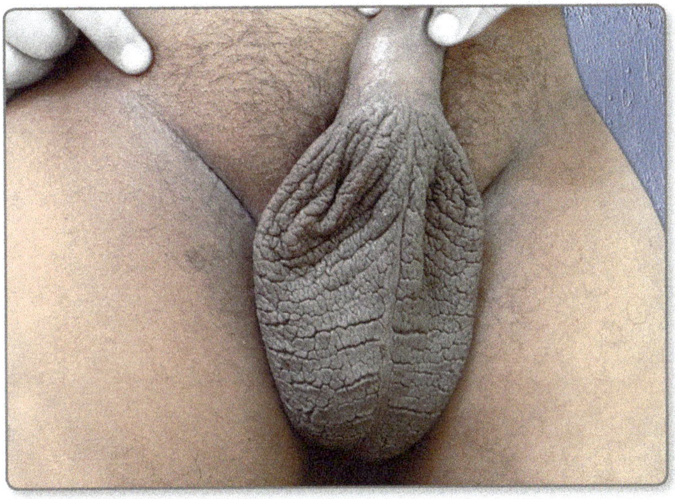

Q. What is the (i) diagnosis and (ii) management?

Answers

i. Scrotal dermatitis.

ii. Management

- To avoid synthetic underwears, strong washing agents for underclothes
- Stress control
- Topical emollients (without fragrances, lanolin, and paraben)
- Topical low potent steroids or tacrolimus or pimecrolimus
- Oral antihistamines.

Case 67

A 25-year-old male had asymptomatic hypopigmented lesions on trunk and limbs for last 3 years mostly aggravating during summer and rainy season. On examination satellite lesions and perifollicular lesions were seen.

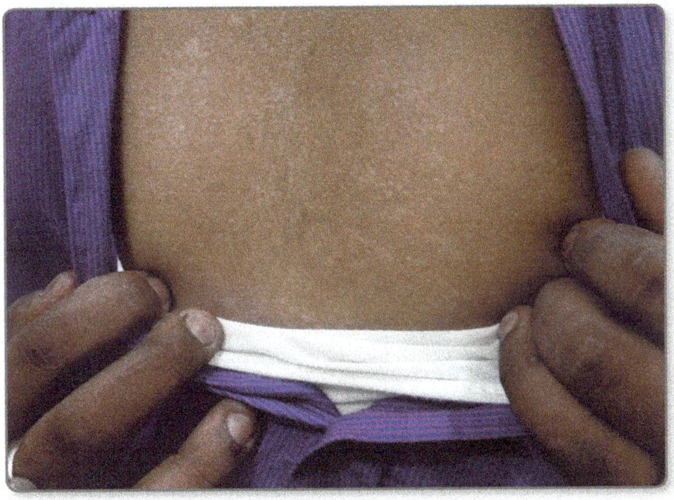

Q. What is the (i) diagnosis and (ii) management?

Answers

i. Pityriasis versicolor.

ii. Management

- Topical 2% ketoconazole shampoo to apply for 5 minutes before bath for 3 consecutive days
- Oral antifungals: Ketoconazole 200 mg daily for 7 days or itraconazole 100–200 mg twice daily for 7 days or fluconazole 400 mg stat.

Case 68

A 3-year-old child had recurrent pruritic popular and papulovesicular lesions mostly on exposed skin (especially both legs and forearms) for last 2 years. On examination many lesions were excoriated.

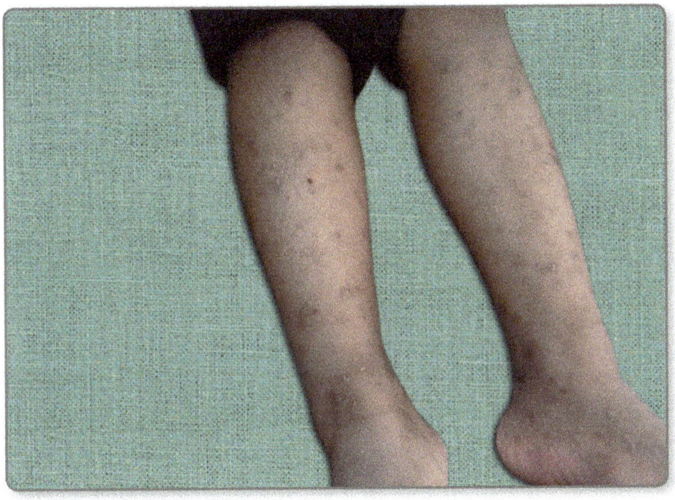

Q. What is the (i) diagnosis and (ii) management?

Answers

i. Papular urticaria.

ii. Management

- To avoid insects (especially mosquito) exposure
- To use full sleeves
- Topical calamine lotion
- Oral antihistamines
- Short course of antibiotics, if secondary infection.

Case 69

A 34-year-old male had recurrent painful boils like swelling on axillae and groins for last 4 years.

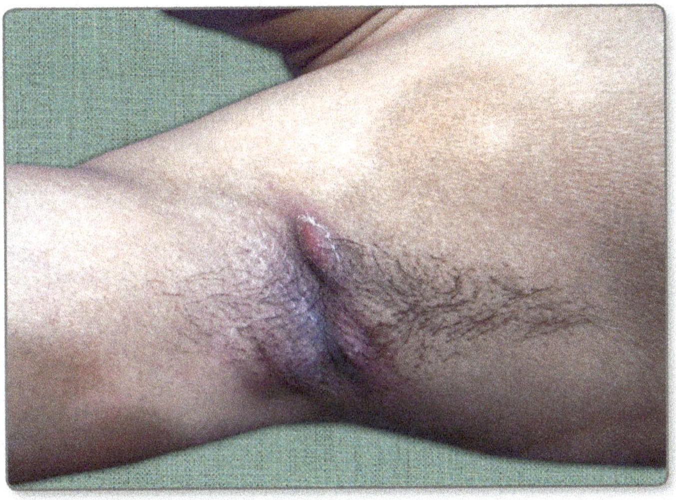

Q. What is the (i) diagnosis and (ii) management?

Answers

i. Hidradenitis suppurativa.

ii. Management

- Weight reduction, loose cloths, avoiding friction, and moisture accumulation
- Topical clindamycin for 3 months
- Systemic tetracycline 250–500 mg 4 times daily until lesions resolved

  or systemic erythromycin 250–500 mg 4 times daily until lesions resolved or oral minocycline 100 mg twice daily until lesions resolved
- Surgery in certain cases.

Case 70

A 6-month-old child had depigmented lesion on abdomen since birth. On examination the lesion sharply demarcated (black arrow) at midline and outer border was bizarre or map-like (blue arrow). On diascopy the lesional border became more distinct.

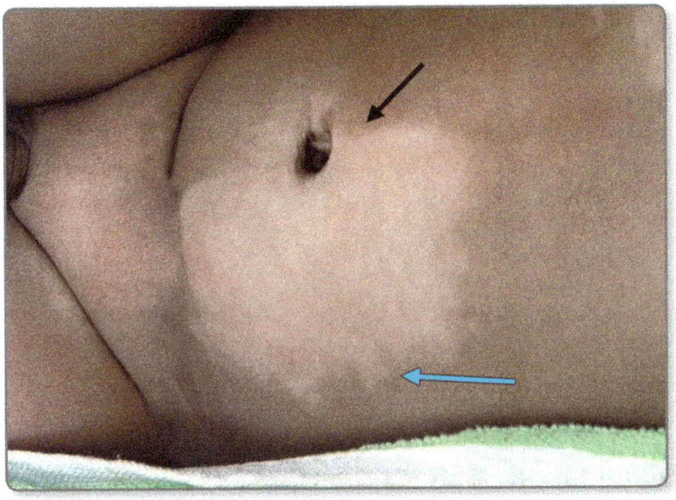

Q. What is the (i) diagnosis and (ii) management?

Answers

i. Nevus depigmentosus.
ii. Management
   - Counseling
   - Watch by mapping
   - Covermark.

Case 71

A 35-year-old male had chronic pruritic lichenified eczematous lesions on palm of the both hands for last 1 year. He had history of contact with cement as construction supervisor.

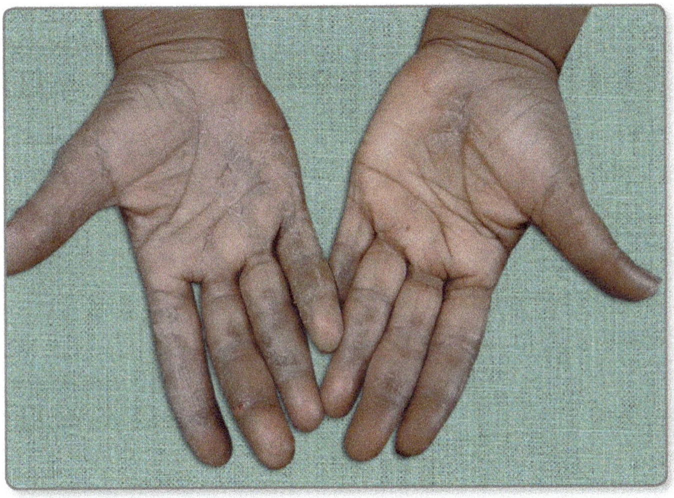

Q. What is the (i) diagnosis and (ii) management?

Answers

i. Contact dermatitis (probably from cement).

ii. Management
- Confirmation of cause of contact dermatitis by allergic patch test
- To use glove/barrier cream while in contact with cement
- Use mild hand wash
- To use emollient liberally
- Potent to super potent topical corticosteroid twice daily followed by mid-potent steroid or tacrolimus ointment
- Oral antihistaminic.

Case 72

A 61-year-old male had asymptomatic depigmented patches on lips, hands and feet for last 5 years which were not progressive.

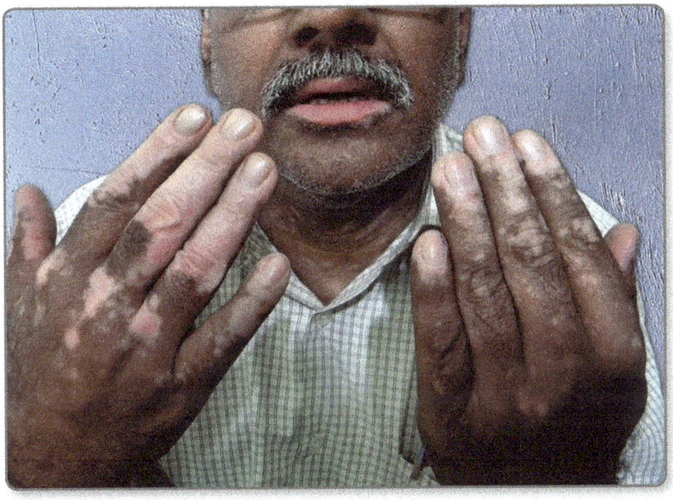

Q. What is the (i) diagnosis and (ii) management?

Answers

i. Vitiligo (lip-tip variety).

ii. Management

- Counseling
- UVB narrow band or PUVA therapy under experienced dermatologist
  or PUVAsol (oral psoralen + sun exposure)
- Covermark.

Case 73

A 18-year-old male had asymptomatic yellowish nodules (black arrow) on elbows and knees for last 2 months. He had family history of dyslipidemia.

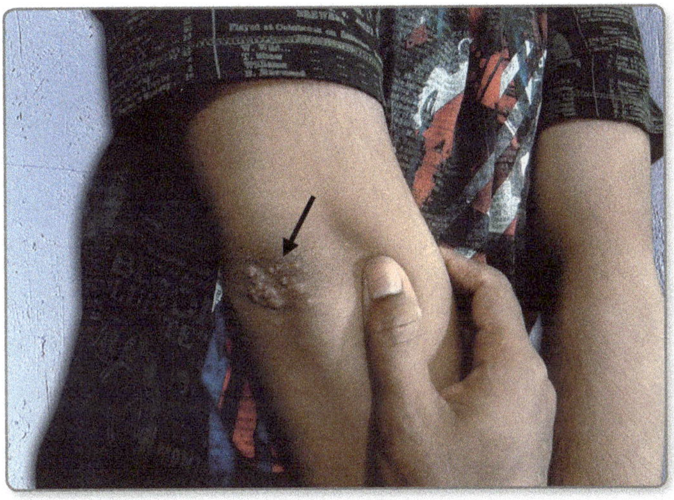

Q. What is the (i) diagnosis and (ii) management?

Answers

i. Eruptive xanthoma.

ii. Management
   - Screening for dyslipidemia
   - Management of dyslipidemia by physician.

Case 74

A 35-year-old lady had multiple asymptomatic umbilicated papules (black arrows) on face for last 3 months. She had history of frequent exposure to beauty parlor for different procedures.

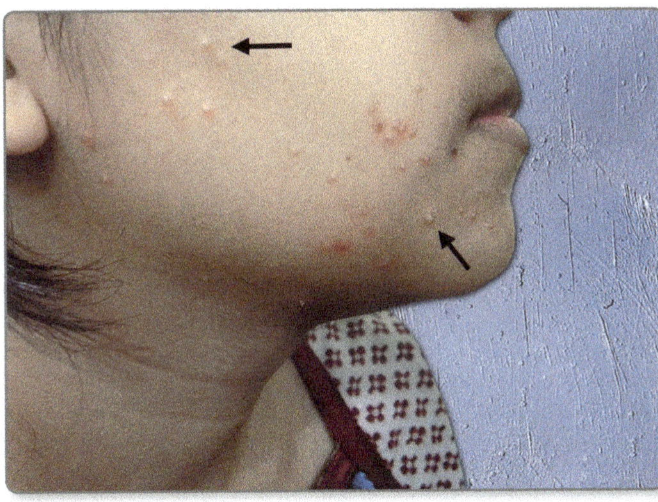

Q. What is the (i) diagnosis and (ii) management?

Answers

i. Molluscum contagiosum.

ii. Management

- Extraction and iodine cautery or light electrofulguration.

Case 75

A 67-year-old male had whitish plaque on glans and prepuce, which had been gradually tightened during 3 years producing acquired phimosis. The patient had also partly narrowing of his urine stream.

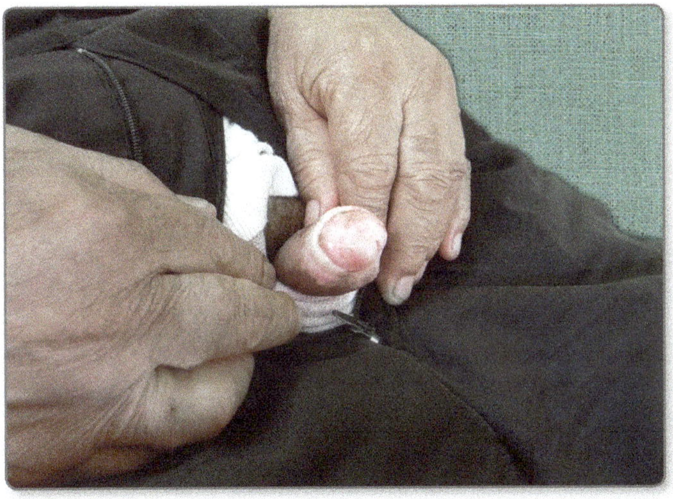

Q. What is the (i) diagnosis and (ii) management?

Answers

i. Lichen sclerosus et atrophicus (LSA) or balanitis xerotica obliterans (BXO).

ii. Management
- Circumscision and biopsy from the glans by urosurgeon
- Urethral dilatation, if needed.

Case 76

A 39-year-old male had nail dystrophy (white arrows) namely, subungual hyperkeratosis, thickening and discoloration of nail plate, on multiple fingers and toes for last 3 years. He had history of diabetes.

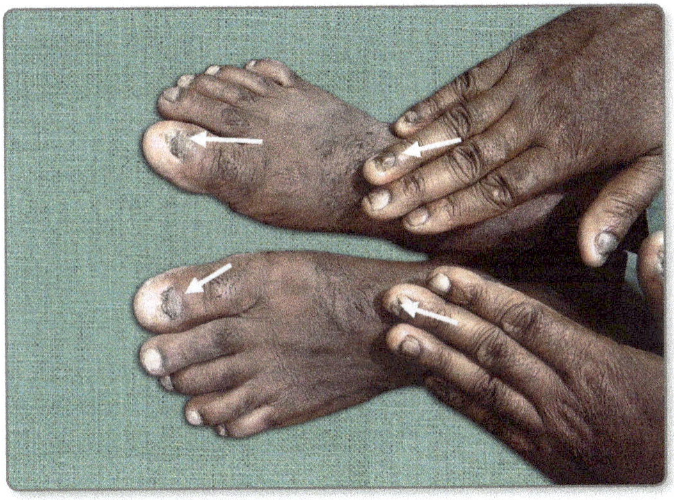

Q. What is the (i) diagnosis and (ii) management?

Answers

i. Tinea unguium or onychomycosis.

ii. Management

- Oral terninafine 250 mg daily for 6 weeks
  or oral itraconazole 200 mg twice daily for 7 days to repeat the pulse for 2 (for fingers) to 3 months (for toes)
  or oral fluconazole 150 mg once in a week for 3 to 6 months
- Topical amorolfine lacquer once in a week for 3 months.

Case 77

A 64-year-old lady suddenly developed frontal baldness for last 6 months. By investigations she had shown high DHEAS level and adrenal tumor by ultrasonography.

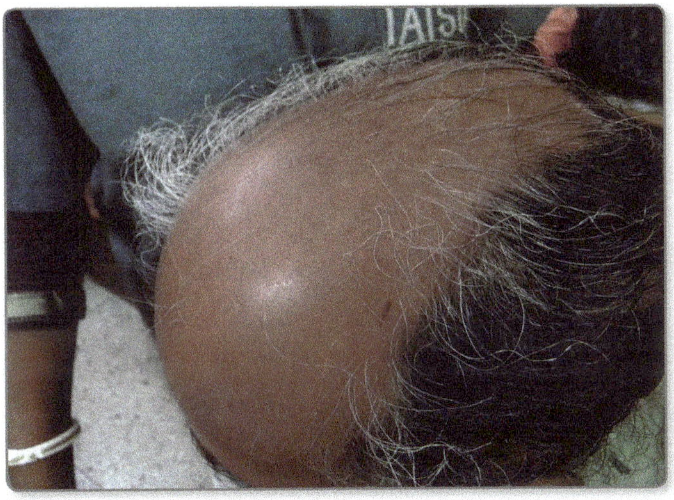

Q. What is the (i) diagnosis and (ii) management?

Answers

i. Androgenetic alopecia due to adrenal tumor.

ii. Management
   - Referral to endocrinologist
   - Topical minoxidil 2% lotion 1 mL twice daily.

Case 78

A 65-year-old male had sudden development of asymptomatic reddish macules and patches on trunk and limbs for last 1 week. On investigations his platelet count was 45,000.

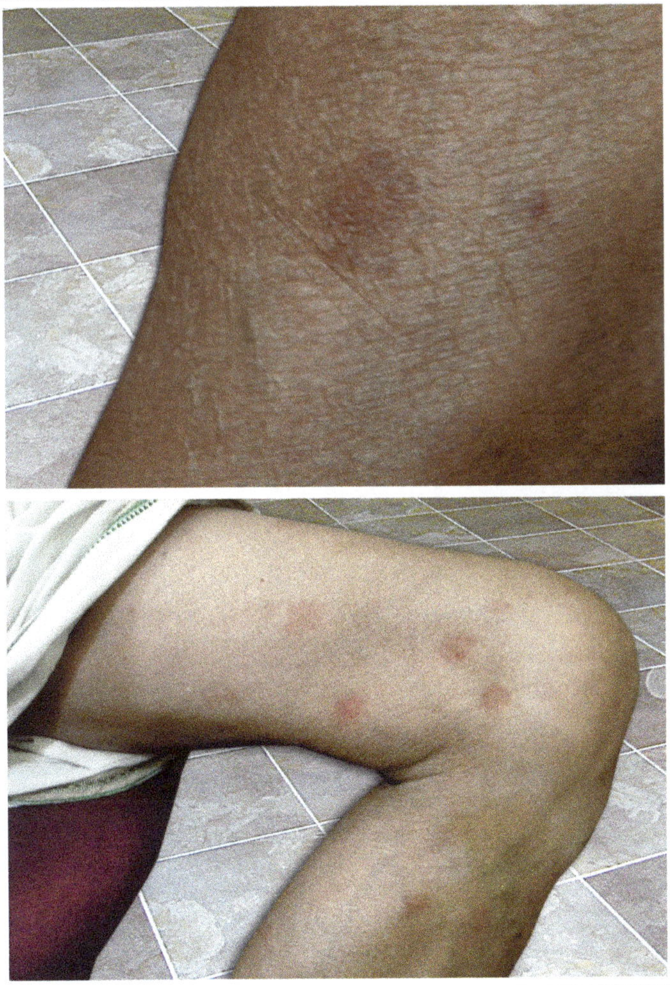

Q. What is the (i) diagnosis and (ii) management?

Answers

i. Thrombocytopenic purpura.

ii. Management
   - Referral to hematologist.

Case 79

A 29-year-old male had mild scaly plaques on scrotum and glans for last 6 months. He had also scaly plaques on elbows, knees and different parts of trunk and nail pitting.

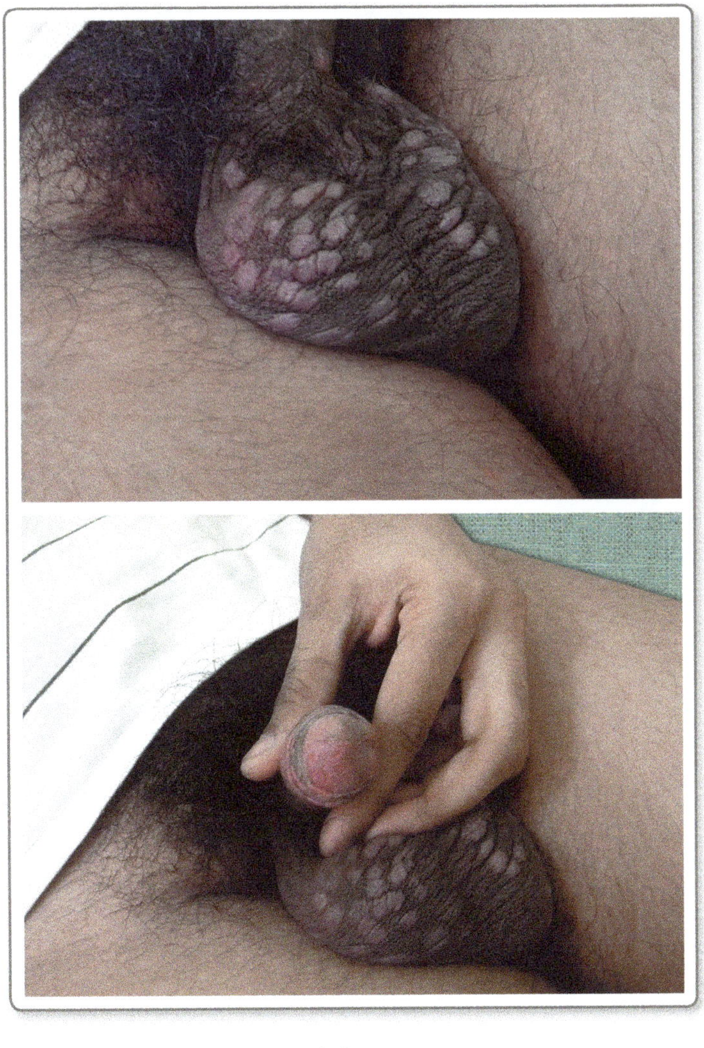

Q. What is the (i) diagnosis and (ii) management?

Answers

i. Psoriasis on scrotum and glans.

ii. Management

- Topical low potent corticosteroid once daily or topical tacrolimus 0.1% or pimecrolimus 1% twice daily.

Case 80

A 23-year-old male had extensive scaly xerotic pruritic lesion almost all over the body for last 3 months. He had history of chronic pruritic flexural dermatitis along with bronchial asthma since childhood. After taking oral steroids for 6 months sudden withdrawal had converted the limited lesions into extensive one.

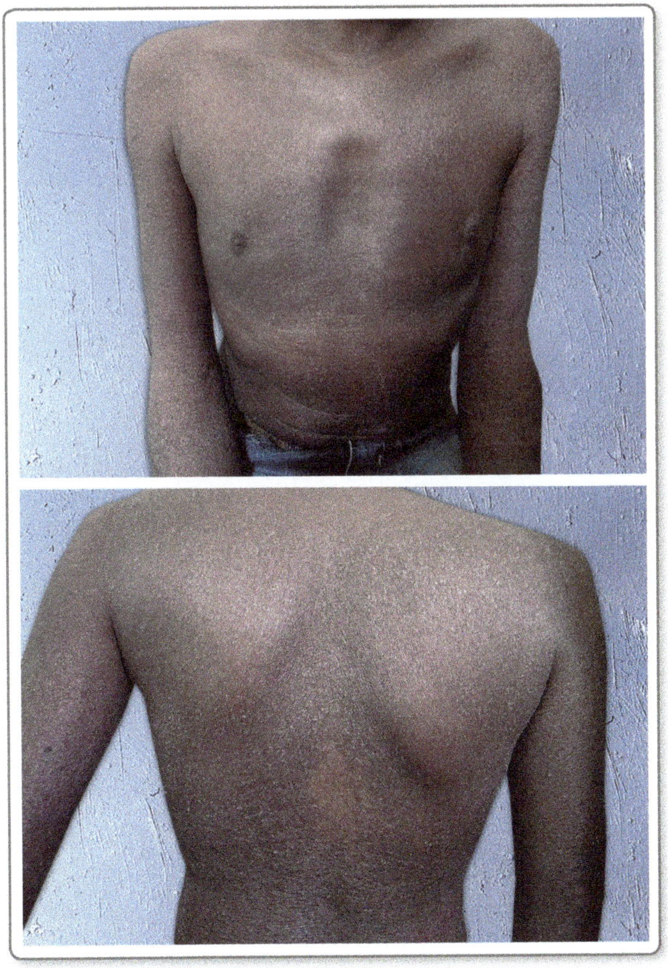

Q. What is the (i) diagnosis and (ii) management?

Answers

i. Exfoliative dermatitis or erythroderma due to atopic dermatitis.

ii. Management
   - Management of erythroderma by admission, fluid-electrolyte and temperature balance, nutrition care, emollient application
   - Treatment of secondary infection
   - Specific treatment of atopic dermatitis: Oral steroids or oral cyclosporine, etc. under expert dermatologist.

Case 81

A 21-year-old female had asymptomatic small scaly (lid-like scale) eruption (blue arrow) followed by hypopigmented patches (black arrow) for last 1 year.

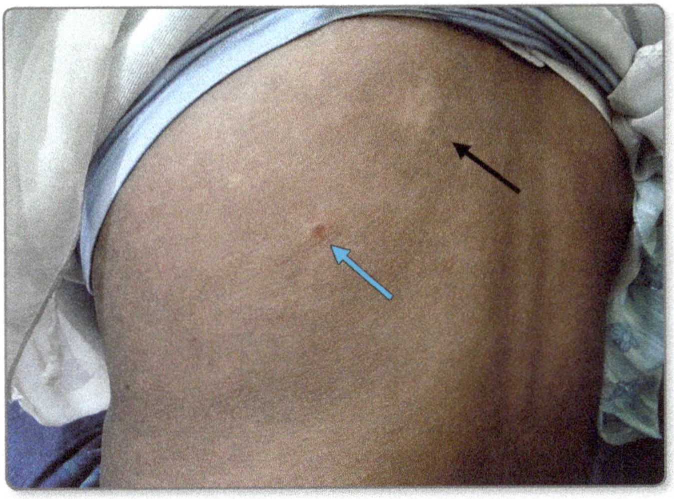

Q. What is the (i) diagnosis and (ii) management?

Answers

i. Pityriasis lichenoid chronica.

ii. Management

- Referral to dermatologist
- UVB NB, PUVA, or PUVAsol therapy
- Topical steroid.

Case 82

A 21-year-old young man had inflammatory papules, pustules and comedones like eruption for last 3 years.

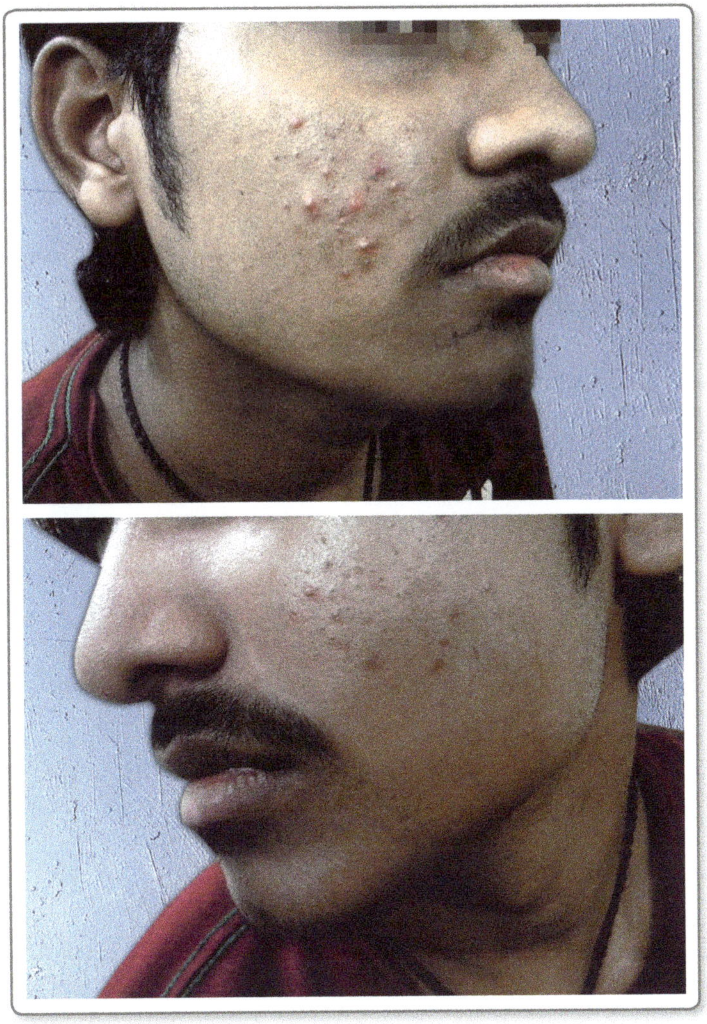

Q. What is the (i) diagnosis and (ii) management?

Answers

i. Acne vulgaris.

ii. Management

- Oral tetracycline 500 mg TID or doxycycline 100 mg daily or minocycline 100 daily up to 3 months
- Topical clindamycin, benzoyl peroxide 2.5% gel or wash, and tretinoin or adapalene.

Case 83

A 34-year-old female had localized scarring alopecia for last 3 years, which was gradually increasing in size. On examination the lesion showed prominent follicular keratosis and atrophy.

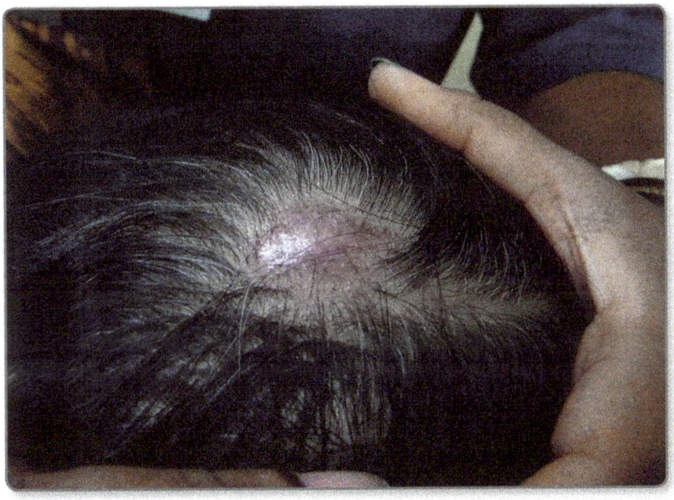

Q. What is the (i) diagnosis and (ii) management?

Answers

i. Cicatrical alopecia due to discoid lupus erythematosus (DLE).

ii. Management

- Avoidance of daylight
- Use of sunscreen/cap/umbrella
- Screening for systemic lupus erythematosus (SLE)
- Oral hydroxychloroquine 200 to 400 mg daily under experienced dermatologist with pre- and per-therapy eye screening.

Case 84

A 31-year-old male had asymptomatic pigmented patches on both axillae for last 6 months. Neither any perifollicular lesion nor any satellite lesions was observed.

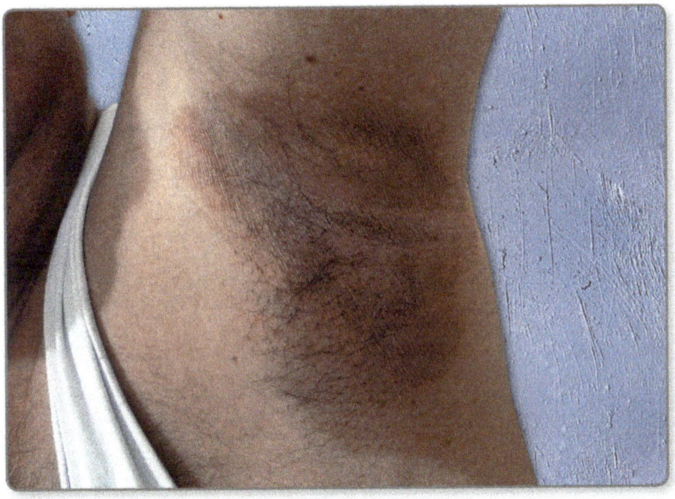

Q. What is the (i) diagnosis and (ii) management?

Answers

i. Erythrasma.

ii. Management
   - Topical benzoyl peroxide 2.5% gel or wash
   - Topical clindamycin or miconazole gel
   - If refractory oral erythromycin 250 mg 4 times daily for 7 days.

Case 85

A 58-year-old lady had chronic eczematous lesions on the tips of her fingers for last 2 years. She had regular habit of contact with different flowers during worship and also different vegetables during cooking.

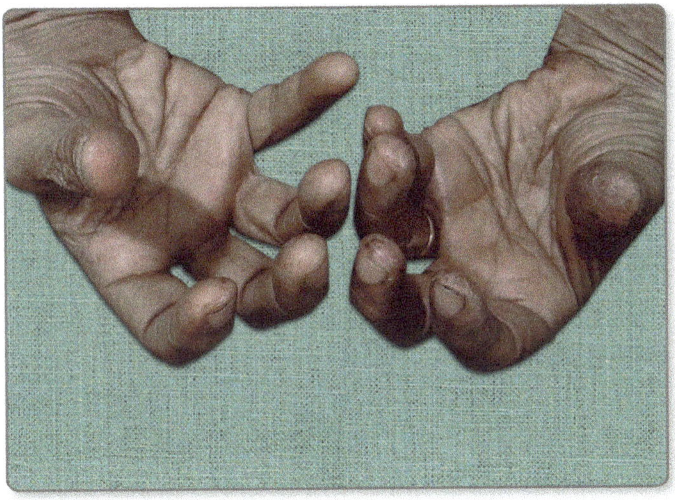

Q. What is the (i) diagnosis and (ii) management?

Answers

i. Contact dermatitis from flowers/vegetables.

ii. Management
  - Avoidance of contact allergens
  - Topical steroids.

Case 86

A 41-year-old lady had asymptomatic pigmented patches (white arrows) on neck, upper chest and back for last 6 months. She was a frequent user of fragrances by spray on neck and upper trunk.

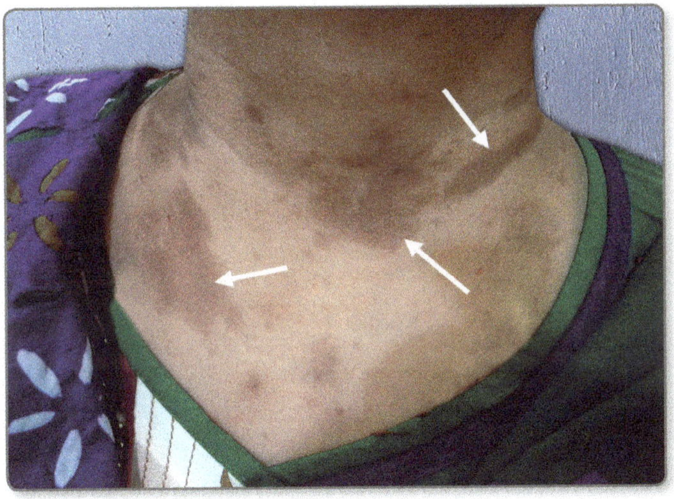

Q. What is the (i) diagnosis and (ii) management?

Answers

i. Pigmented contact dermatitis from fragrances.

ii. Management
  - Avoidance of fragrances
  - Topical steroids
  - Broad spectrum sunscreen.

Case 87

A 65-year-old male had sudden loss of hair for last 2 months producing circumscribed area of alopecia, which did not show any scarring.

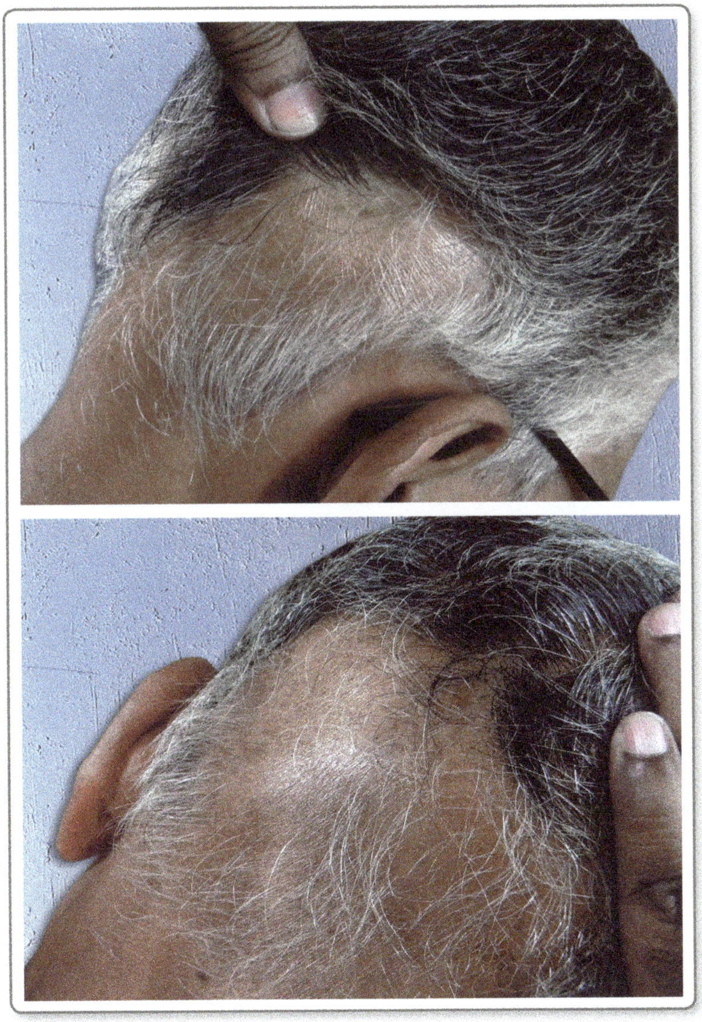

Q. What is the (i) diagnosis and (ii) management?

Answers

i. Alopecia areata.

ii. Management

- Topical super potent corticosteroid or intralesional triamcinolone by expert dermatologist
- If refractory, contact immunotherapy.

Case 88

A 38-year-old female had painful hyperkeratotic lesions (black arrows) on different parts of the feet for last 5 years. On examination the lesions were more tender on ventral pressure than lateral pressure.

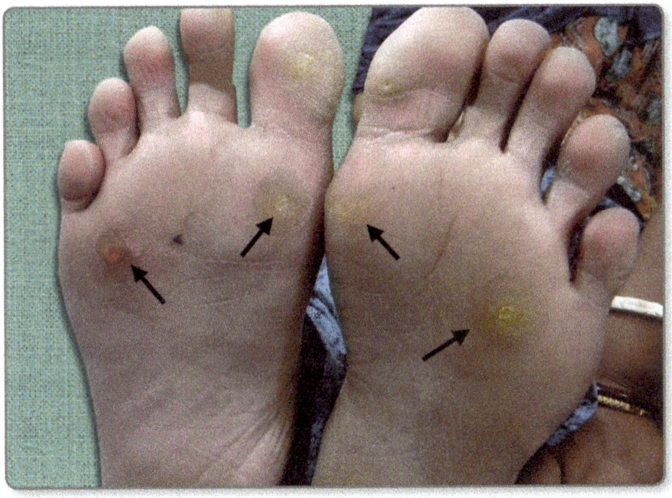

Q. What is the (i) diagnosis and (ii) management?

Answers

i. Plantar corn (callosity).

ii. Management

- Proper shoe
- Salicylic acid 16.5%
- Lactic acid 16.5%
- Collodion flexile 25 mL
- Mft pig
- Apply at night with applicator only on corns.

Case 89

A 46-year-old lady had chronic dry lesions (black arrows) on palms especially in between fingers for last 3 years. She had history of frequent water and soap wash of hands.

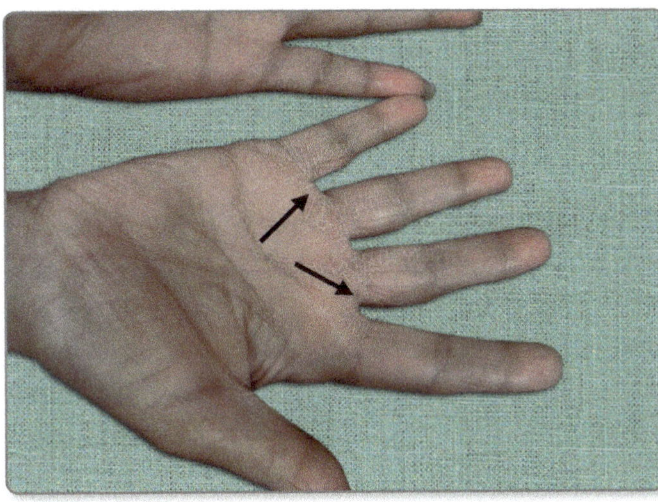

Q. What is the (i) diagnosis and (ii) management?

Answers

i. Irritant contact dermatitis (chronic cumulative).
ii. Management
   - Restricted soap and water use
   - Liberal use of emollients
   - Topical potent steroids.

Case 90

A lady had chronic erosion on tongue for last 5 years, which on examination, showed erythematous raw area with loss of papillae and sharp whitish circinate or serpiginous border.

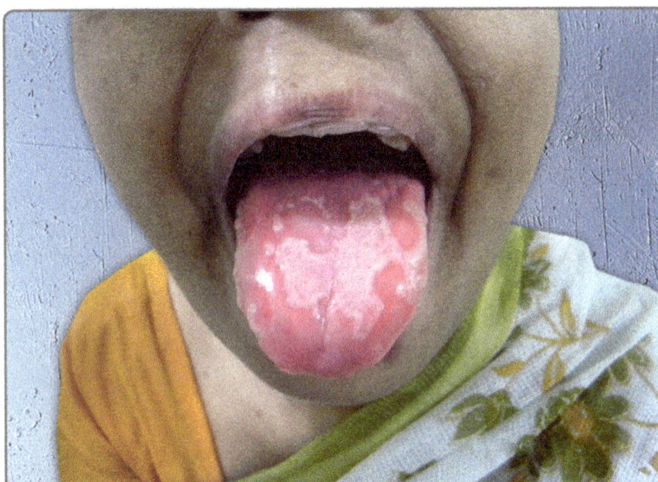

Q. What is the (i) diagnosis and (ii) management?

Answers

i. Geographic tongue
ii. Management
  - Counseling
  - Topical lignocaine for pain relieve
  - Clotrimazole troche to suck twice daily to control secondary candidiasis.

Case 91

A 31-year-old lady had asymptomatic thick yellowish plaques on both eyelids for last 1 year. She had family history of similar lesions.

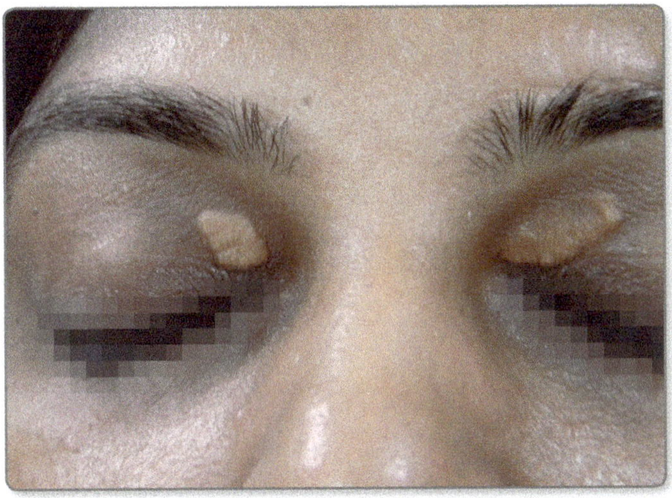

Q. What is the (i) diagnosis and (ii) management?

Answers

i. Xanthelasma palpebrarum.

ii. Management

- Screening serum lipid profile
- Counseling
- Topical TCA application by expert dermatologist.

Case 92

A 51-year-old female had asymptomatic pigmented patches on both cheeks for last 2 years.

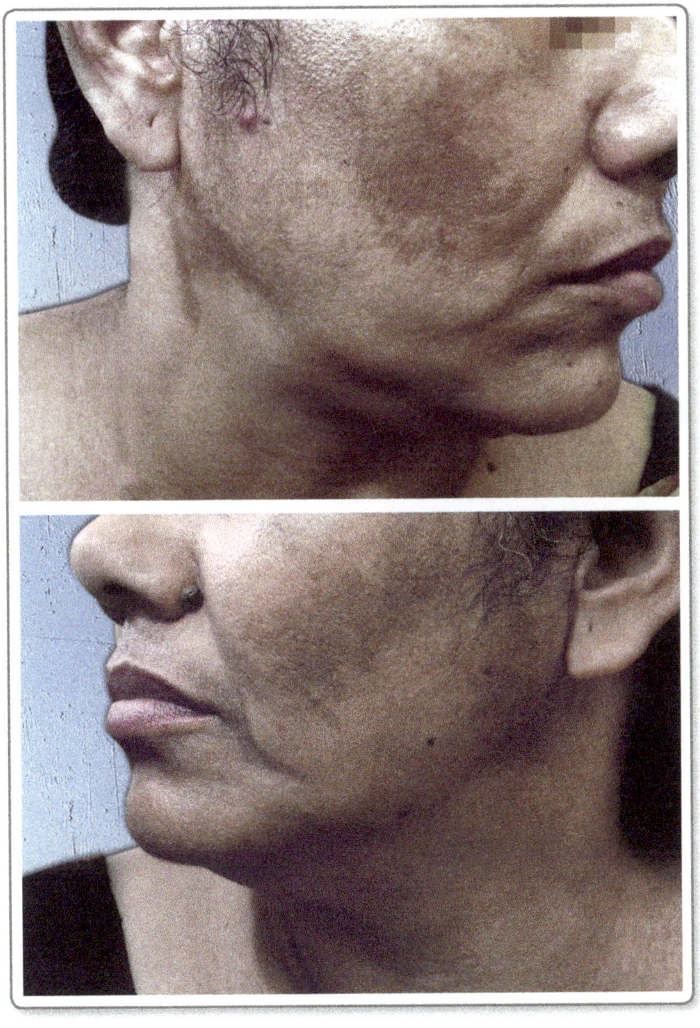

Q. What is the (i) diagnosis and (ii) management?

Answers

i. Melasma.

ii. Management

- Broad spectrum sunscreen
- Topical hydroquinone 2%, tretinoin 0.025% or topical kozic acid 2% or glycolic acid 6%
- For short period topical low potent steroid can be used.

Case 93

A 29-year-old lady had papulovesicular eruptions on both forearms, V-area of neck, and back of neck for last 2 weeks at the end of the spring. She had similar eruptions at same sites during same time last 2 years.

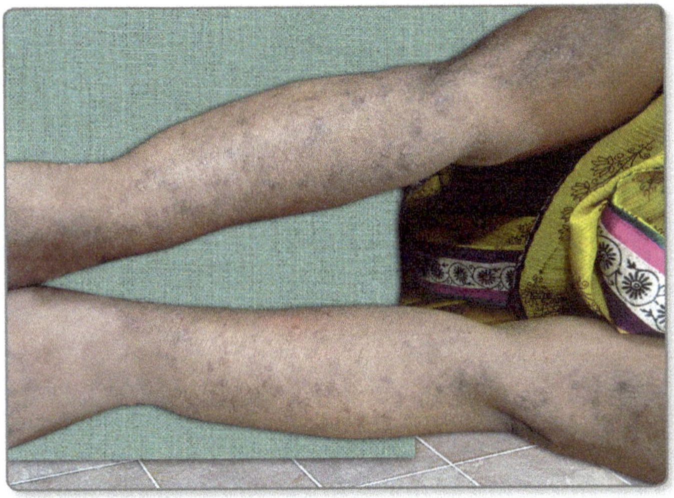

Q. What is the (i) diagnosis and (ii) management?

Answers

i. Polymorphous light eruption.
ii. Management
   - Avoidance of daylight
   - Topical mid-potent steroids
   - Antihistamines
   - Broad spectrum sunscreen.

Case 94

A 51-year-old lady had superficial pustular eruptions often in annular distribution mostly in intertriginous area (axillae, inframammary, and groin) for last 5 years.

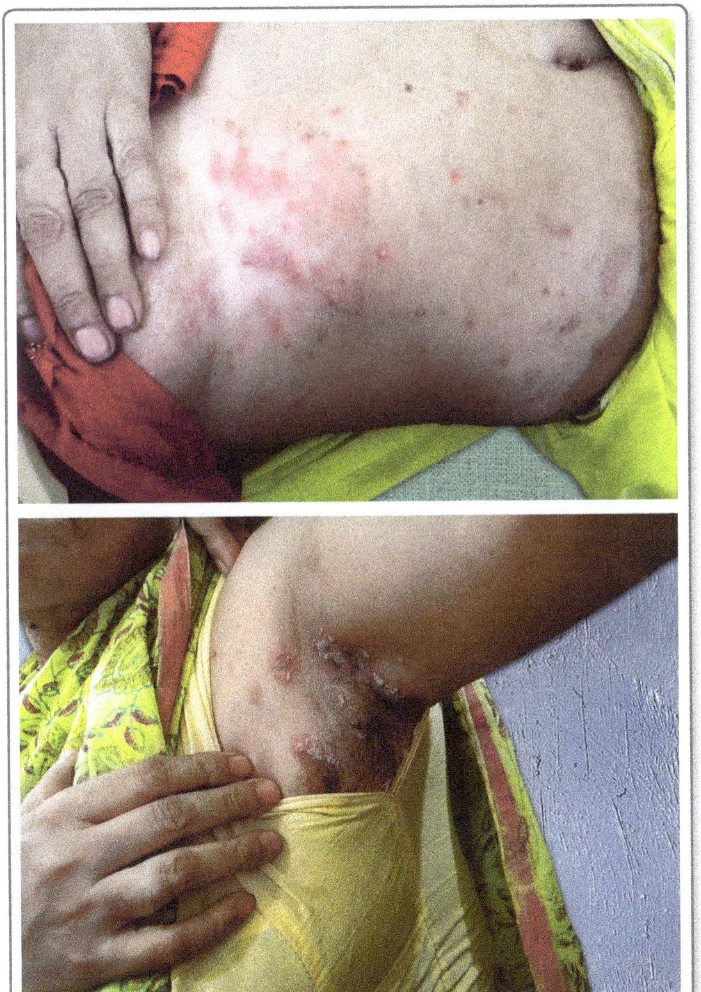

Q. What is the (i) diagnosis and (ii) management?

Answers

i. Subcorneal pustular dermatoses (SCPD).
ii. Management
   - Referral to competent dermatologist
   - Confirmation by histopathology test
   - Dapsone under dermatologist's supervision by previous G-6 PD screening (quantitative).

Case 95

A 31-year-old male had extensive papulosquamous skin eruption involving scalp, eyelids, postauricular region, front of the chest and back (interscapular region) and groin for last 5 years.

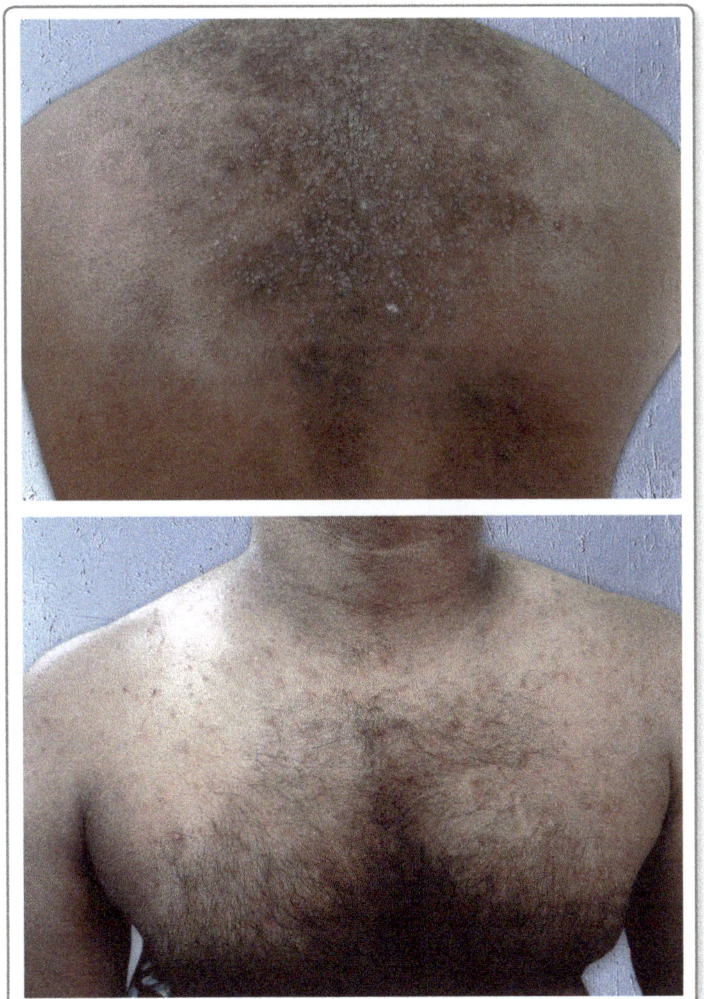

Q. What is the (i) diagnosis and (ii) management?

Answers

i. Seborrheic dermatitis

ii. Management

- Avoidance of oil/oily lotion
- Oral tetracycline/doxycycline
- Topical antifungal-steroid combination.

Case 96

A 28-year-old lady had history of tick-bite followed by a progressively increased annular lesion with trail-like margin on left calf for last 6 weeks. She had no history of fever, arthralgia, cardiac, or neurological symptom.

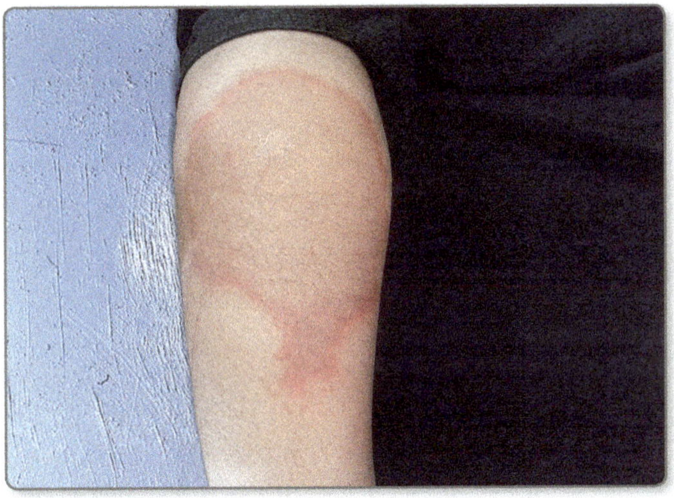

Q. What is the (i) diagnosis and (ii) management?

Answers

i. Erythema migrans.

ii. Management

- Screening for systemic symptoms of borreliosis
- Oral doxycycline 100 mg twice daily for 3 weeks
  or oral erythromycin 250 mg 4 times daily for 3 weeks.

Case 97

A 34-year-old female had erythematous pruritic eruption on face, neck and forearms for last 5 months. Her submental area was not spared (white arrows). She had been contact with cement dust during her profession of construction supervisor.

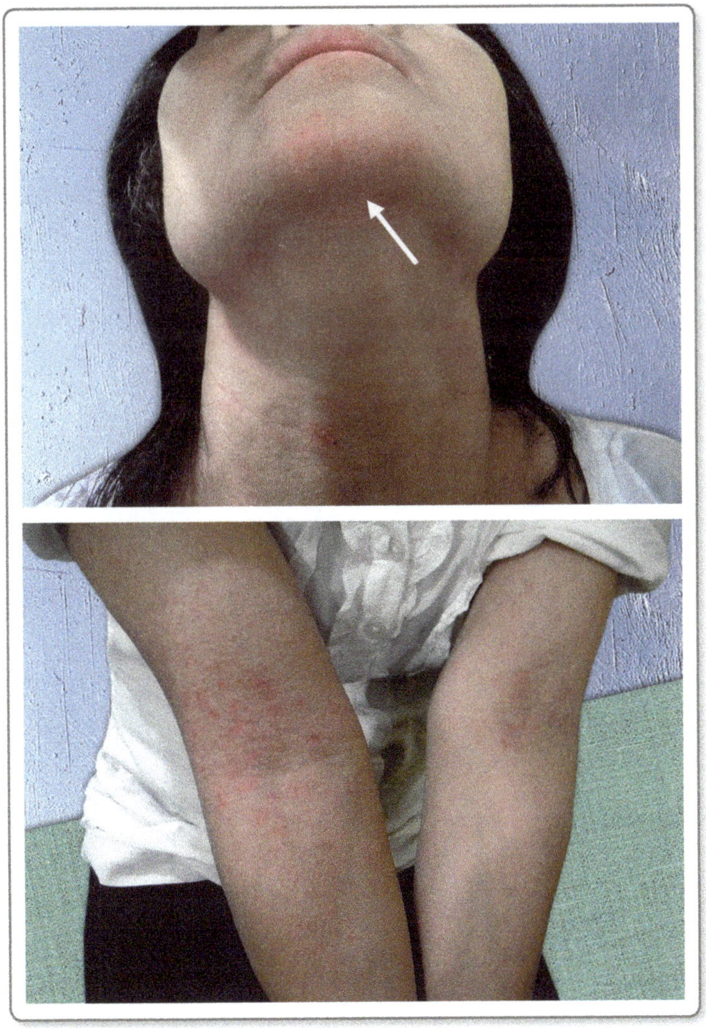

Q. What is the (i) diagnosis and (ii) management?

Answers

i. Airborne contact dermatitis to cement dust (potassium dichromate) (in photoallergic contact dermatitis or PACD submental area is spared).

ii. Management
   - To avoid cement dust as far as possible by using full sleeves, etc.
   - Topical low potent steroid or tacrolimus on face
   - Topical potent steroid on trunk and limbs
   - Antihistamines
   - Oral short course steroid, if refractory.

Case 98

A 32-year-old male had sudden development of depigmented patch surrounding a pigmented mole during last 3 months

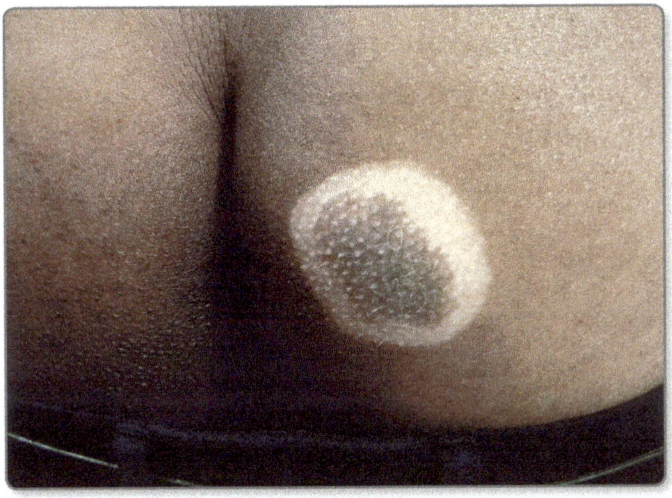

Q. What is the (i) diagnosis and (ii) management?

Answers

i. Halo nevus.

ii. Management

- Topical tacrolimus 0.1% twice daily or topical steroid once daily
- In refractory case, total excision of the mole.

Case 99

A 31-year-old lady had itchy, scaly annular lesions on lower abdomen, waist and left foot for last 3 months. The lesions had active inflammatory border with central clearing.

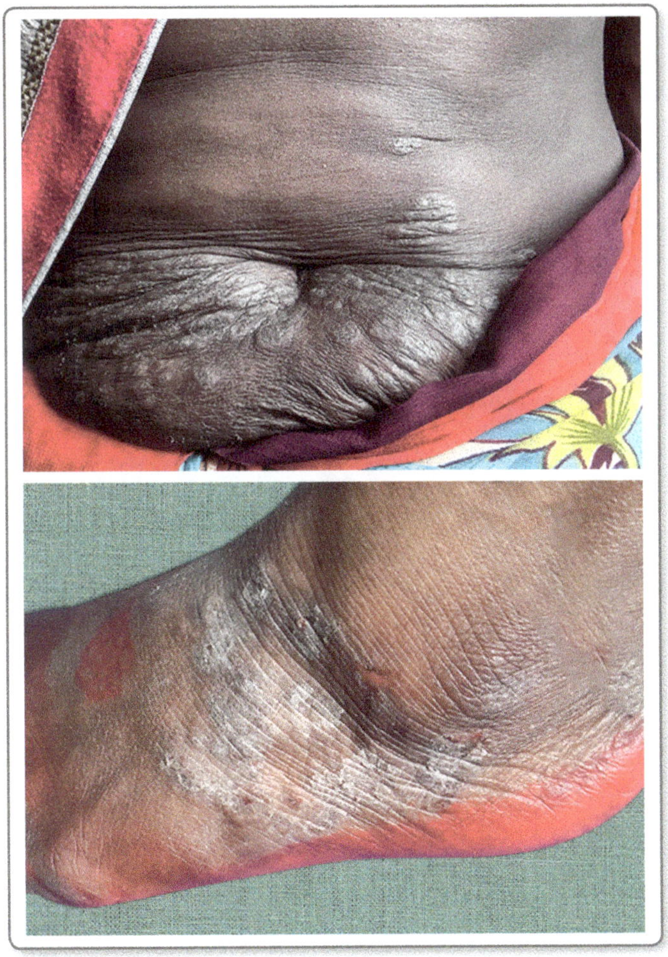

Q. What is the (i) diagnosis and (ii) management?

Answers

i. Tinea corporis.

ii. Management

- Oral terbinafine 250 OD for 15 days
  or, oral fluconazole 150 mg once/week for 4 weeks
  or, oral itraconazole 100 mg BD for 14 days
- Topical terbinafine, sertaconazole, luliconazole, or amorolfine daily for 4 weeks.

Case 100

A 52-year-old female had asymptomatic pigmented macules and patches on lower legs and feet for last 2 years.

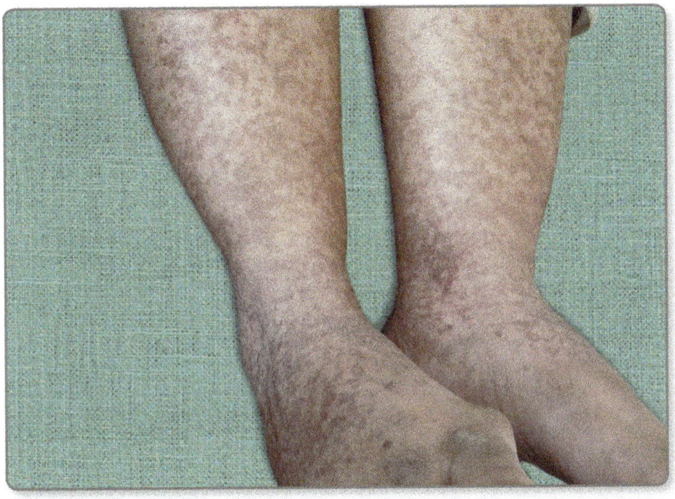

Q. What is the (i) diagnosis and (ii) management?

Answers

i. Pigmented purpuric dermatoses (PPD).
ii. Management
   - To rule out underlying venous stasis
   - To avoid prolonged standing
   - Potent topical steroids.

Case 101

A 14-year-old male had chronic eczematous lesion on left foot for last 6 months. He had started the ailment after wearing a new 'chappal.'

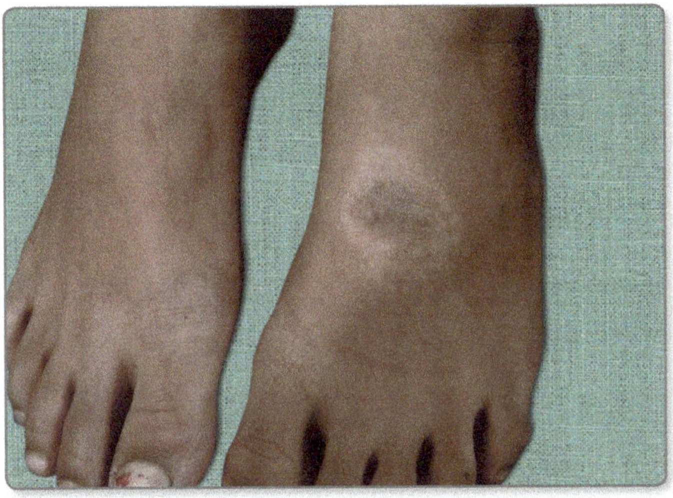

Q. What is the (i) diagnosis and (ii) management?

Answers

i. Allergic contact dermatitis from footwear (may be unilateral).

ii. Management

- Confirmation and detection of exact allergen of footwear by allergic patch test
- Avoidance of relevant allergens
- Topical corticosteroid.

Case 102

A 13-year-old boy had recurrent pruritic vesicles on palm and feet for last 4 years.

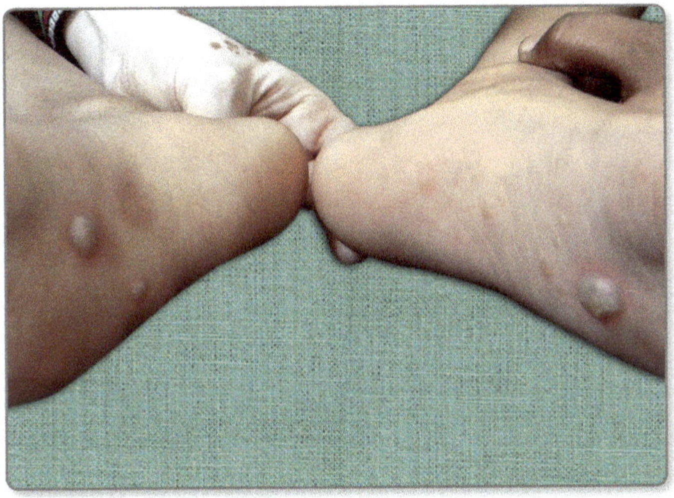

Q. What is the (i) diagnosis and (ii) management?

Answers

i. Vesicular dermatitis of hands and feet (pompholyx).
ii. Management
   - To detect any associated fungal infection or eczematous lesions or septic focus inside body
   - Topical corticosteroid
   - Oral antihistamines.

Case 103

A 34-year-old male had recurrent intertriginous eruption on groin (black arrow) for last 5 years which mostly aggravated during winter. He had also thick hyperkeratotic lesions (white arrow) on knees and elbows.

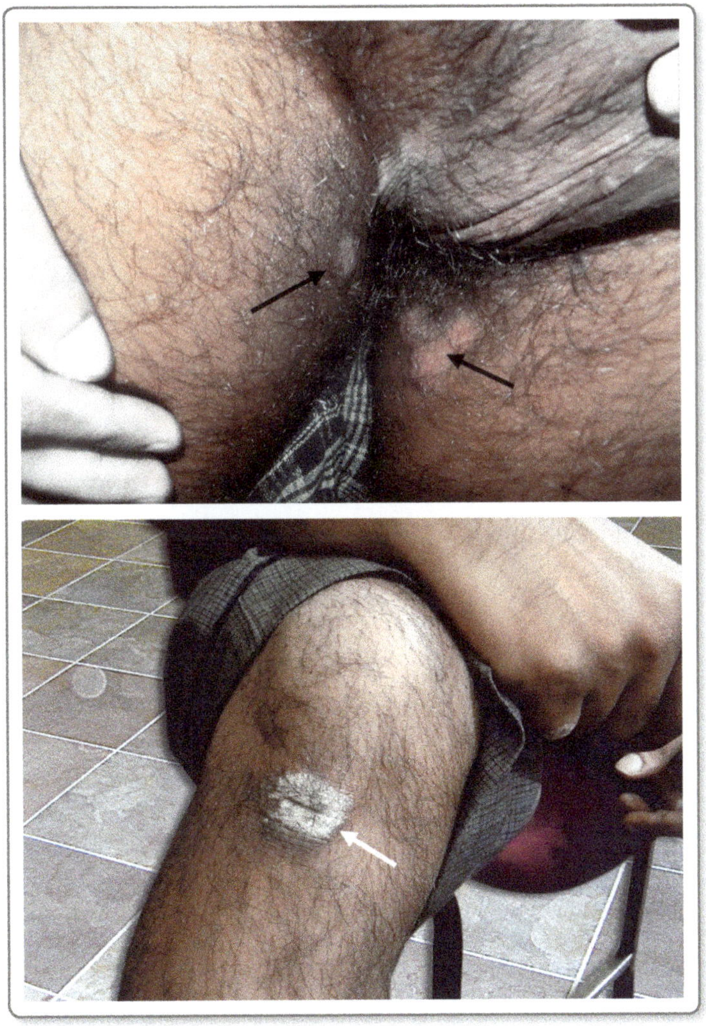

Q. What is the (i) diagnosis and (ii) management?

Answers

i. Flexural (inverse) psoriasis with chronic plaque psoriasis.

ii. Management

- Topical tacrolimus 0.03–0.5% or pimecrolimus 1% twice daily on groin patches
- Management of chronic plaque psoriasis as per body surface area (BSA) involvement.

Case 104

A 26-year-old female had chronic pruritic plaques for last 3 years. She had also oral lacy pattern of lesions for last 4 years.

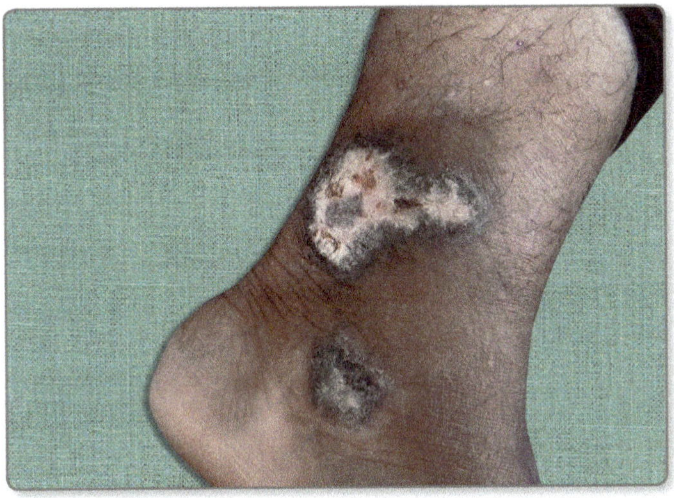

Q. What is the (i) diagnosis and (ii) management?

Answers

i. Lichen planus hypertrophicus.

ii. Management

- Super potent topical steroid by monitoring
- Intralesional triamcinolone by expert dermatologist
- Oral antihistamines.

Case 105

A 41-year-old male had well-circumscribed hyperkeratotic lesions on feet for last 5 years mostly aggravating in winter. He had nail pitting and well-defined scaly plaques on scalp.

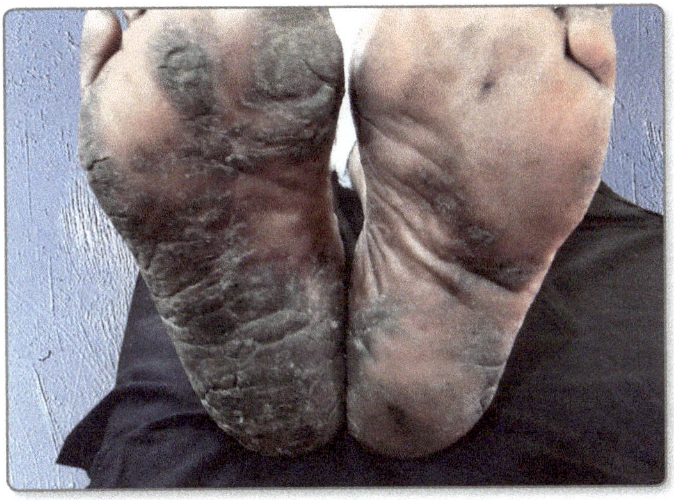

Q. What is the (i) diagnosis and (ii) management?

Answers

i. Plantar psoriasis.

ii. Management
- Topical super potent corticosteroid with or without 3% salicylic acid
- Topical tar or dithranol (short contact)
- If refractory, PUVA or methotrexate under expert dermatologist.

Case 106

A 26-year-old male had sudden onset maculopapular eruption on trunk, limbs and palms and sole for last 5 days. He had history of oral amoxycillin 1 week back for throat infection.

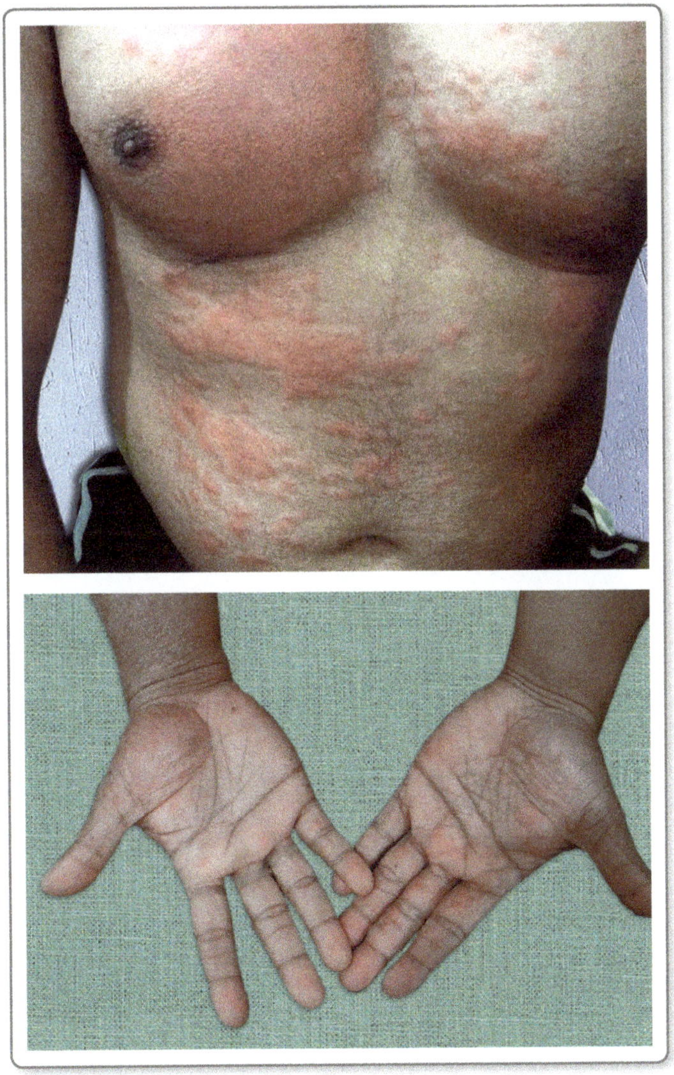

Q. What is the (i) diagnosis and (ii) management?

Answers

i. Adverse cutaneous drug eruption (maculopapular).

ii. Management
- Strict avoidance of relevant drugs and cross-reactants
- Monitoring for systemic involvement
- Topical corticosteroid lotion or cream
- Oral antihistamines
- Short course of oral steroids, if severe.

Case 107

A 23-year-old female had distal separation of left great toe nail for last 4 months. On examination the color of the nail (arrow) appeared greenish.

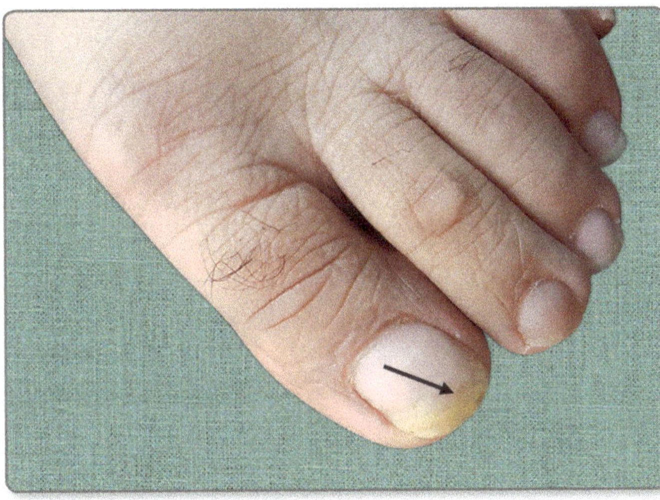

Q. What is the (i) diagnosis and (ii) management?

Answers

i. Tinea unguium or onychomycosis.

ii. Management

- Oral terbinafine 250 OD for 6 weeks
  or, oral fluconazole 150 mg once/week for 3 to 6 months
  or, oral itraconazole 200 mg twice daily for 7 days, then to repeat the pulse twice for finger nails and thrice for toe nails (once in a month)
- Topical amorolfine or ciclopirox lacquer once in a week for 3 months.

Case 108

A 68-year-old male had well-defined scaly erythematous plaques on different area of trunk (periumbilical, pubic area, etc.) and extensor surface of limbs. The scale were loose, white and scraping the scales lead to bleeding (Auspitz sign positive).

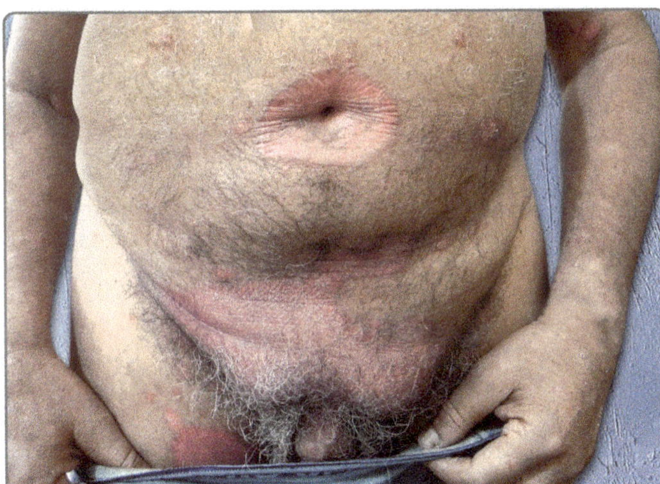

Q. What is the (i) diagnosis and (ii) management?

Answers

i. Psoriasis vulgaris (chronic plaque).

ii. Management

- Topical emollient
- Topical low potent steroid
- UVB narrow band or PUVA
- If refractory: Oral methotrexate or injection etanercept by screening and monitoring.

Case 109

A 31-year-old male had warty lesion on glans (black arrow) for last 6 months. He had history of extramarital sexual exposure.

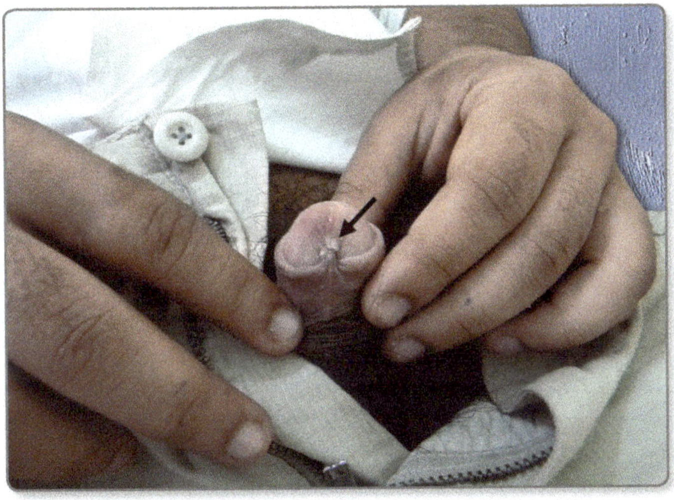

Q. What is the (i) diagnosis and (ii) management?

Answers

i. Condyloma acuminata.

ii. Management

- Screening for other STDs, especially HIV
- Imiquimod 5% thrice in a week
- Cryosurgery or electrosurgery under expert dermatologist.

Case 110

A 31-year-old male had extensive hyperpigmented scaly lesions on trunk and limbs for last 2 months in summer. He had similar eruption in last 3 years during summer. On examination, the eruption had satellite lesions and perifollicular distribution.

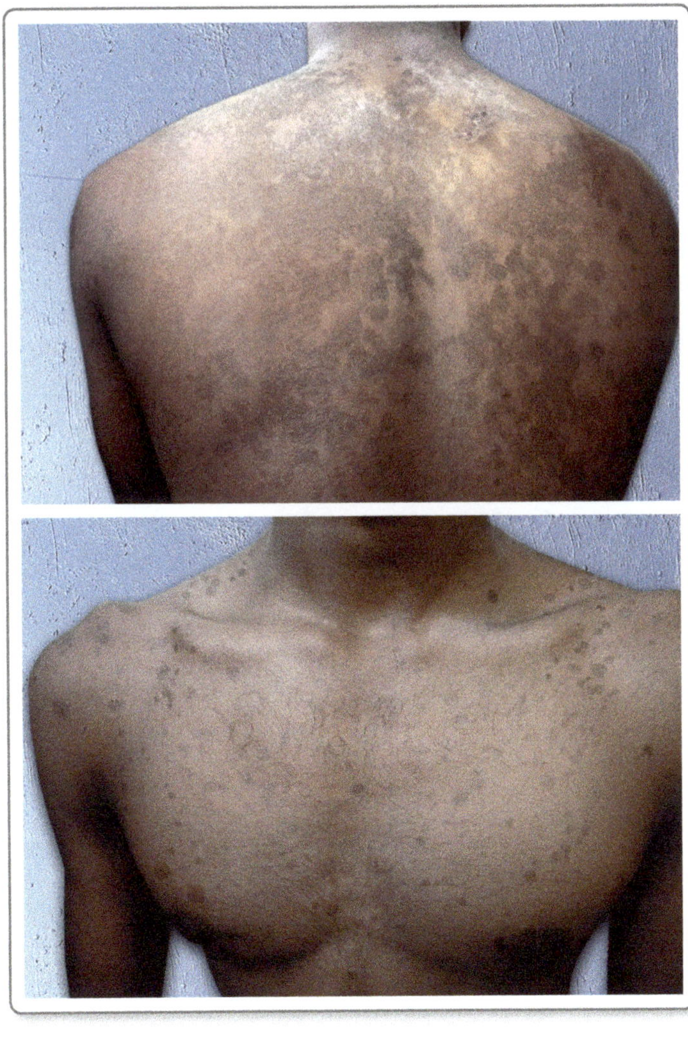

Q. What is the (i) diagnosis and (ii) management?

Answers

i. Pityriasis versicolor.

ii. Management
  - Topical 2% ketoconazole shampoo to apply for 5 minutes before bath for 3 consecutive days
  - Oral antifungals: Ketoconazole 200 mg daily for 7 days or itraconazole 100–200 mg twice daily for 7 days or fluconazole 400 mg stat.

Case 111

A 31-year-old lady had pruritic erythematous papular and pustular eruption on face for last 6 months. She had history of intermittent application of potent topical steroid for last 3 years.

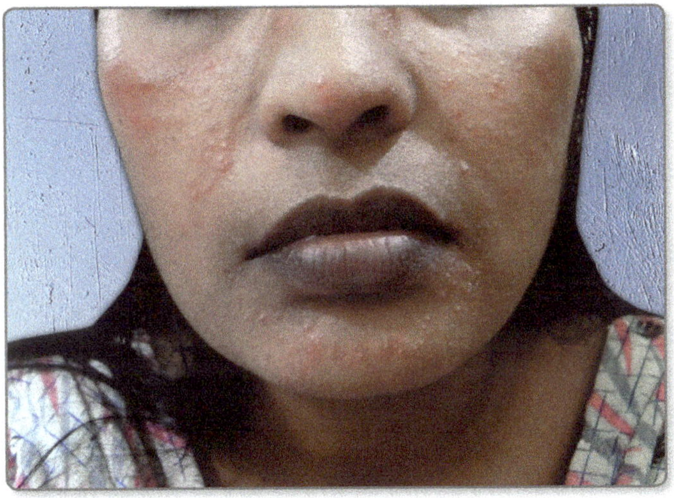

Q. What is the (i) diagnosis and (ii) management?

Answers

i. Iatrosacea due to topical steroid.

ii. Management

- Topical low potent steroid to be gradually tapered off and to be followed by topical tacrolimus 0.03–0.1% or pimecrolimus twice daily
- If refractory: Oral tetracycline, doxycycline or minocycline.

Case 112

A 36-year-old male had recurrent painful boils-like eruption (black arrow) on scalp for last 2 years.

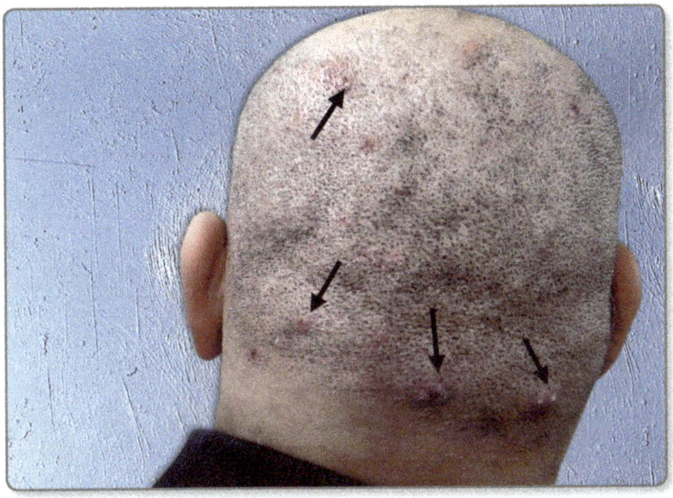

Q. What is the (i) diagnosis and (ii) management?

Answers

i. Folliculitis decalvans.

ii. Management

- Oral tetracycline or doxycycline or minocycline for long-term
- Topical retapamulin, mupirocin, or fucidic acid
- Povidone iodine shampoo.

Case 113

A 64-year-old male had gradual onset bullous eruption which were tense and hemorrhagic (black arrow) during last 6 months. He had no oral mucosal lesion.

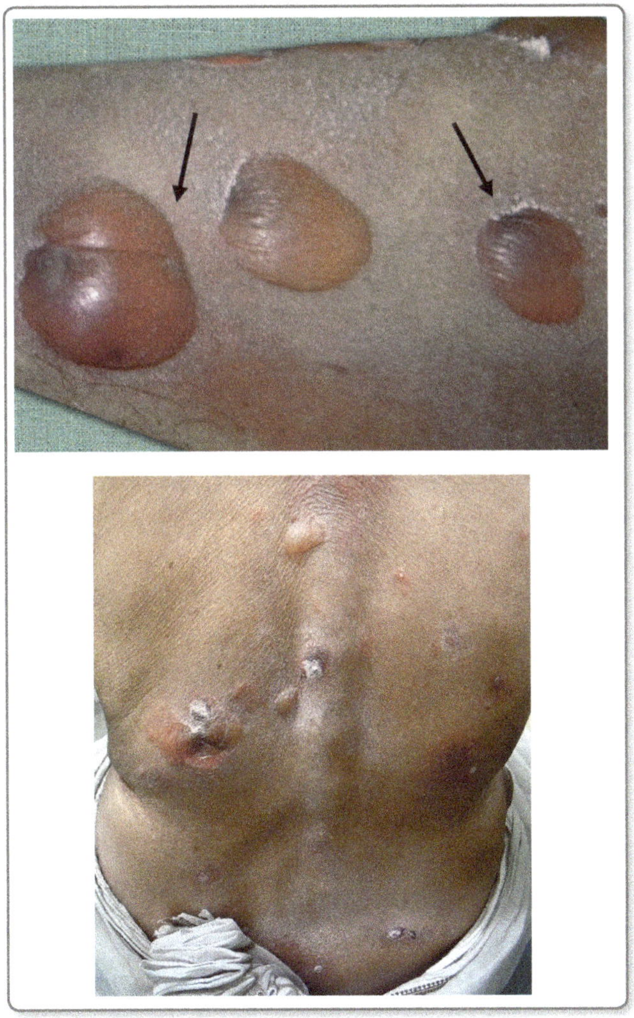

Q. What is the (i) diagnosis and (ii) management?

Answers

i. Bullous pemphigoid.

ii. Management
   - Confirmation of diagnosis by skin biopsy
   - Oral corticosteroid and adjuvant (azathioprine, mycophenolate mofetil, etc.) under expert dermatologist by strict monitoring.

Case 114

A 65-year-old lady had sudden onset pain in left ear and left side of face followed by grouped vesicular eruption in dermatomal distribution (black arrow) and external ear (blue arrow) for last 3 days.

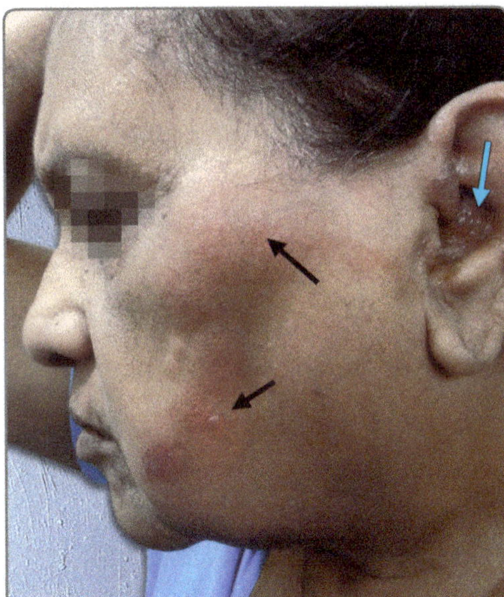

Q. What is the (i) diagnosis and (ii) management?

Answers

i. Herpes zoster oticus (Ramsay Hunt syndrome).
ii. Management
   - Referral to ENT surgeon to manage for facial palsy, if any
   - Oral valacyclovir 1,000 mg thrice daily or acyclovir 800 mg 5 times daily or famciclovir 500 mg thrice daily for 7 days.

Case 115

A 23-year-old male had multiple painful hard noduloulcerative lesions on glans and prepuce for last 1 week. He had associated painful lymphadenopathy. He had history of exposure to a sexual-worker.

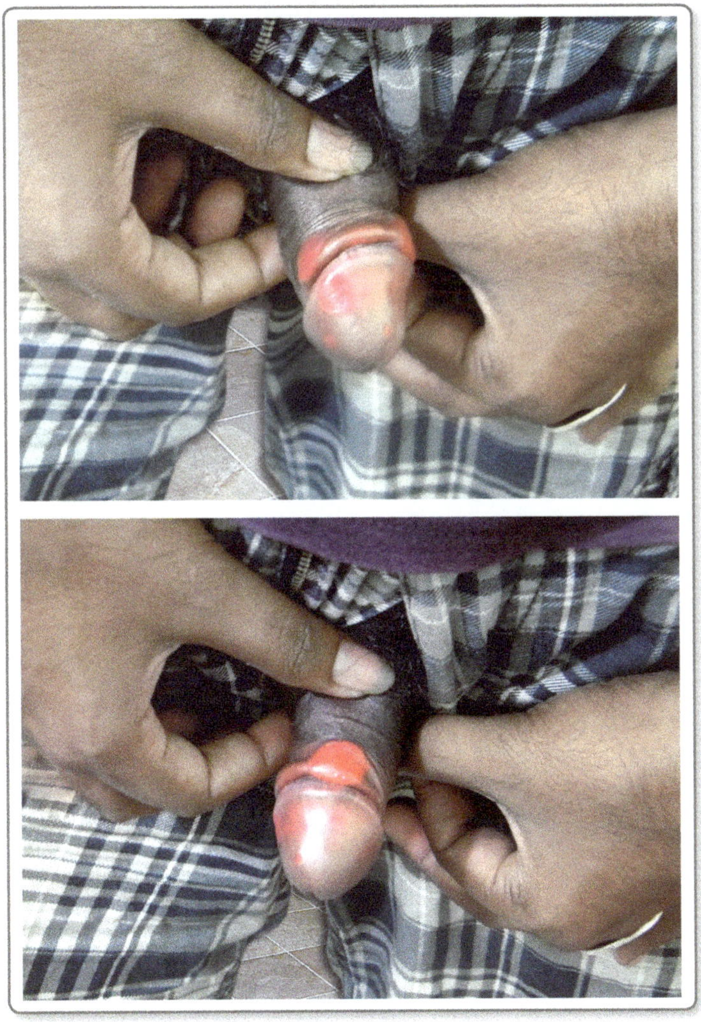

Q. What is the (i) diagnosis and (ii) management?

Answers

i. Chancroid.

ii. Management

- Screening for other STDs, especially HIV
- Azithromycin 1 g single dose
  or ceftriaxone 250 mg IM single dose
  or ciprofloxacin 500 mg BID for 3 days
  or erythromycin 500 mg 4 times daily for 7 days.

Case 116

A 49-year-old male had coppery colored hypoesthetic patches on right elbow and right side of abdomen (black arrows) for last 6 months. Right radial nerve was thickened but not tender.

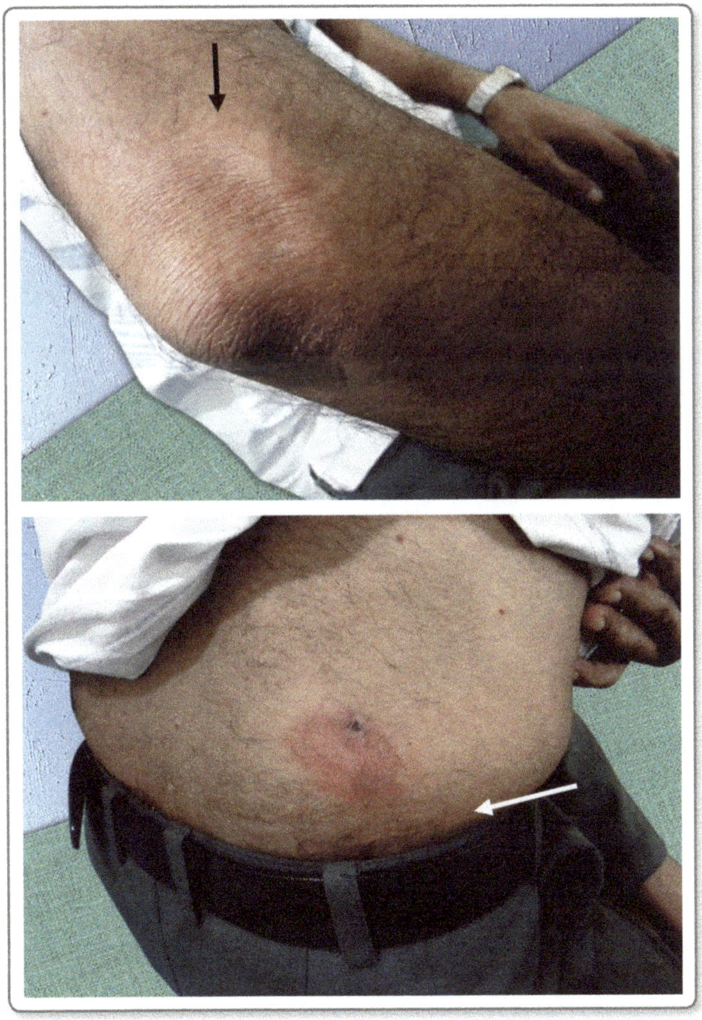

Q. What is the (i) diagnosis and (ii) management?

Answers

i. Hanseniasis (paucibacillary: Borderline tuberculoid [BT]).

ii. Management

- Dapsone 100 mg daily
- Rifampicin 600 mg orally once in empty stomach (supervised).

Case 117

A 26-year-old lady had generalized pustular eruption (black arrow) and lake of pus (blue arrow) with fever for last 3 months. She had previous history of psoriasis vulgasis and been treated with oral corticosteroids.

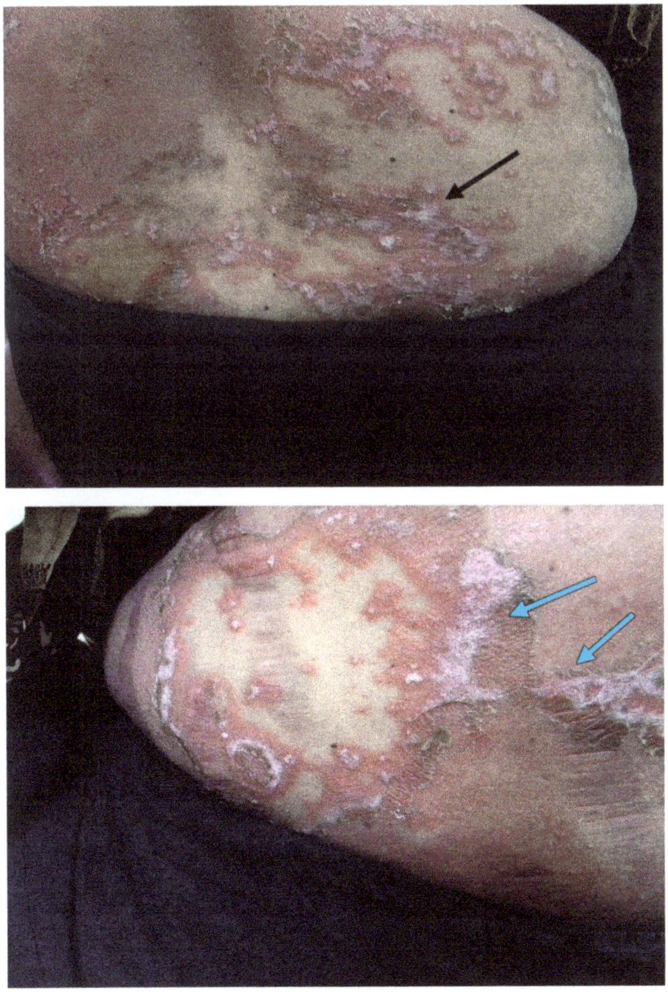

Q. What is the (i) diagnosis and (ii) management?

Answers

i. Pustular psoriasis.
ii. Management
   - Admission under dermatologist and internist
   - Oral cyclosporin under expert dermatologist.

Case 118

A 31-year-old lady had recurrent acneiform eruption around mouth for last 8 months. She had history of application of topical corticosteroid and lot of cosmetics.

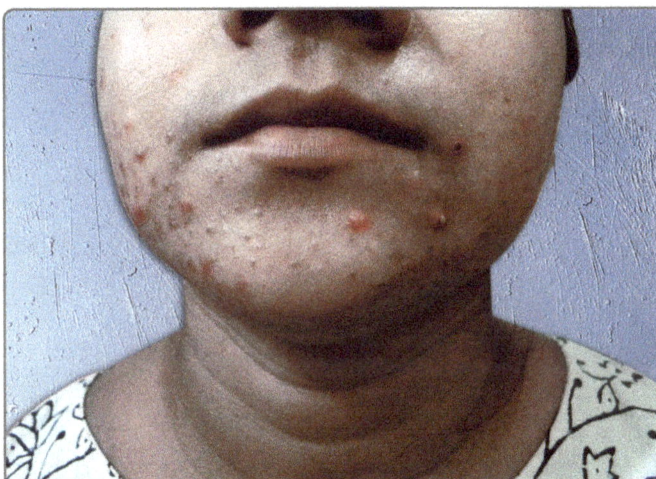

Q. What is the (i) diagnosis and (ii) management?

Answers

i. Perioral dermatitis.

ii Management

- Oral tetracycline or doxycycline
- Topical clindamycin or benzoyl peroxide.

Case 119

A 35-year-old male had multiple umbilicated papules around genitalia for last 5 months. He had extramarital partner.

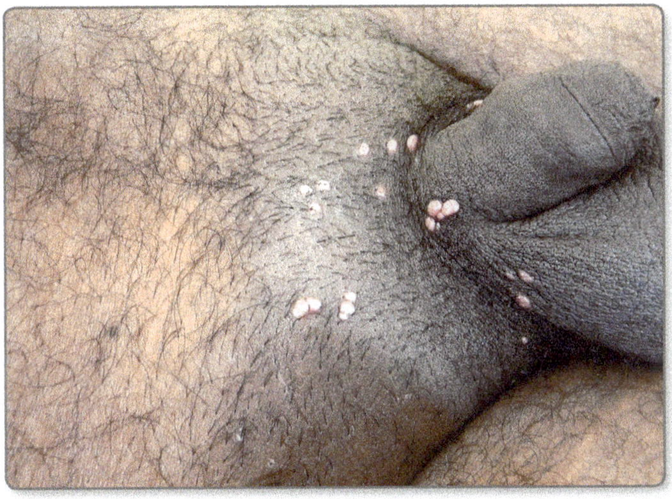

Q. What is the (i) diagnosis and (ii) management?

Answers

i. Molluscum contagiosum (perigenital).

ii. Management
  - Screening for other STDs, especially HIV
  - Extraction and chemical cautery, or electrosurgery, or cryosurgery.

Case 120

A 23-year-old female had multiple discharging ulcers with underlying lymphadenopathy on left side of neck for last 1 year. She had history of low grade fever, cough, night sweating, and loss of weight.

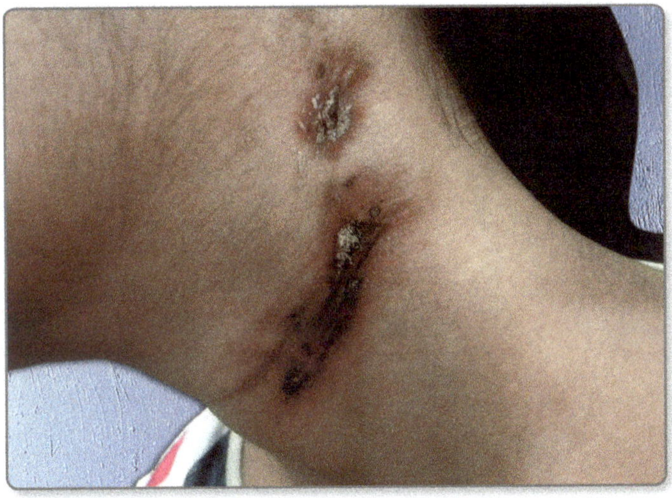

Q. What is the (i) diagnosis and (ii) management?

Answers

i. Scrofuloderma.

ii. Management

- Referral to tuberculosis specialist and surgeon
- Confirmation of diagnosis
- Full antituberculous regimen under tuberculosis specialist.

Case 121

A 4-month-old female infant had extensive eczematous eruption on extensor aspect of limbs, face and trunk for last 1 month. She had history of bronchial spasm and family history of asthma and eczema.

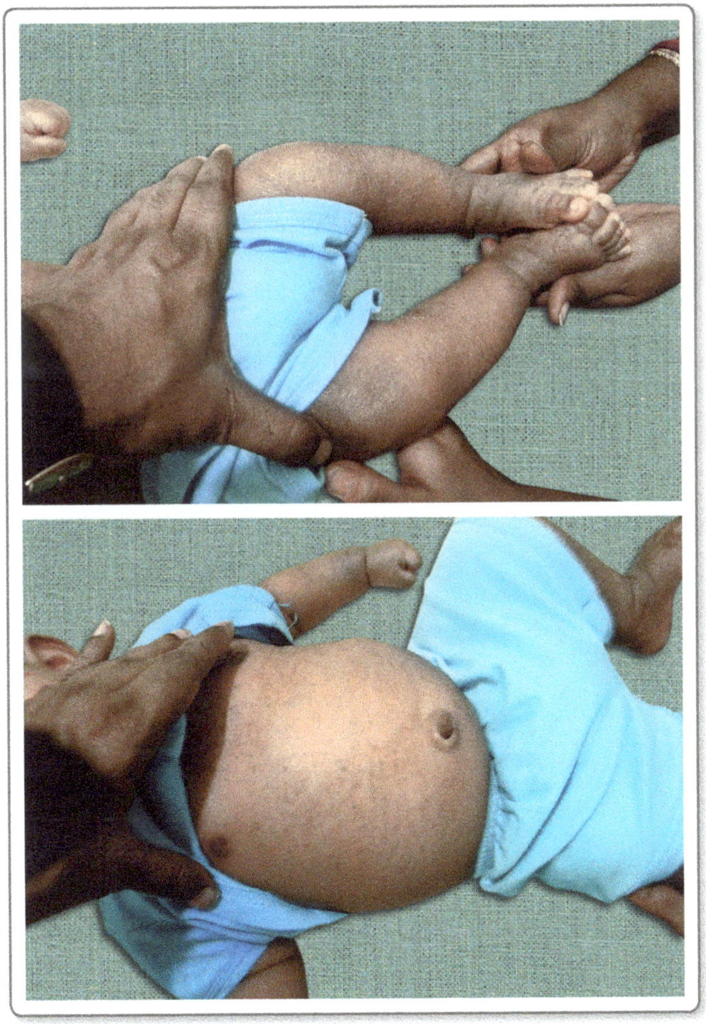

Q. What is the (i) diagnosis and (ii) management?

Answers

i. Atopic dermatitis (*in infants extensor aspect involved compared to flexural involvement in older children*).

ii. Management
   - Topical emollients
   - Low potent topical steroid
   - Avoidance of atopic triggers.

Case 122

A 52-year-old female had extensive pruritic eruption with complaints of some insects always crawling on her skin for last 3 years. She brought some dead insect-like objects in a plastic container. She expressed history of disharmony with her daughter-in-law.

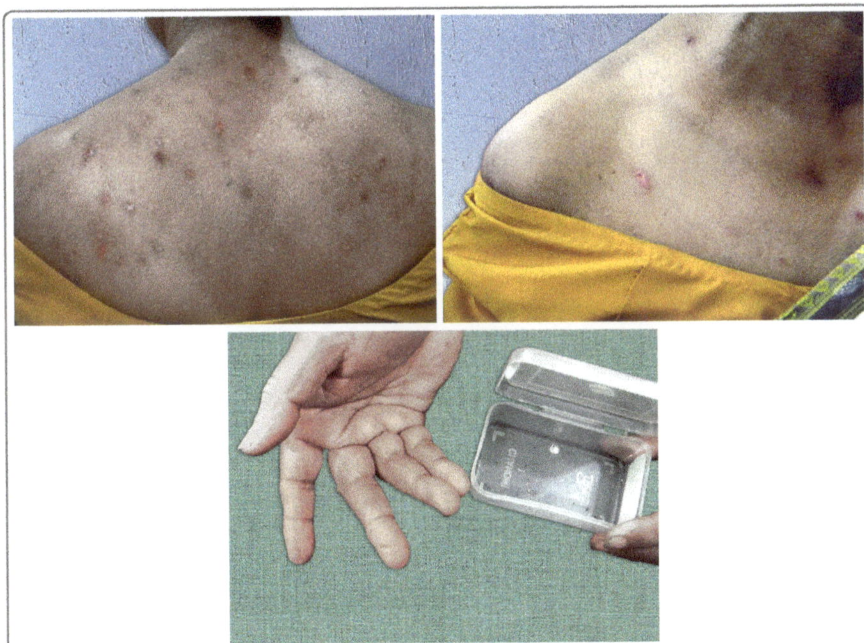

Q. What is the (i) diagnosis and (ii) management?

Answers

i. Delusion of parasitosis.

ii. Management
   - Referral to psychiatrist
   - Topical calamine to relieve itching.

Case 123

A 24-year-old female had malar flush, photosensitivity, oral ulceration on hard palate, skin eruption on photo-exposed skin alongwith fever, and arthralgia for last 1 year.

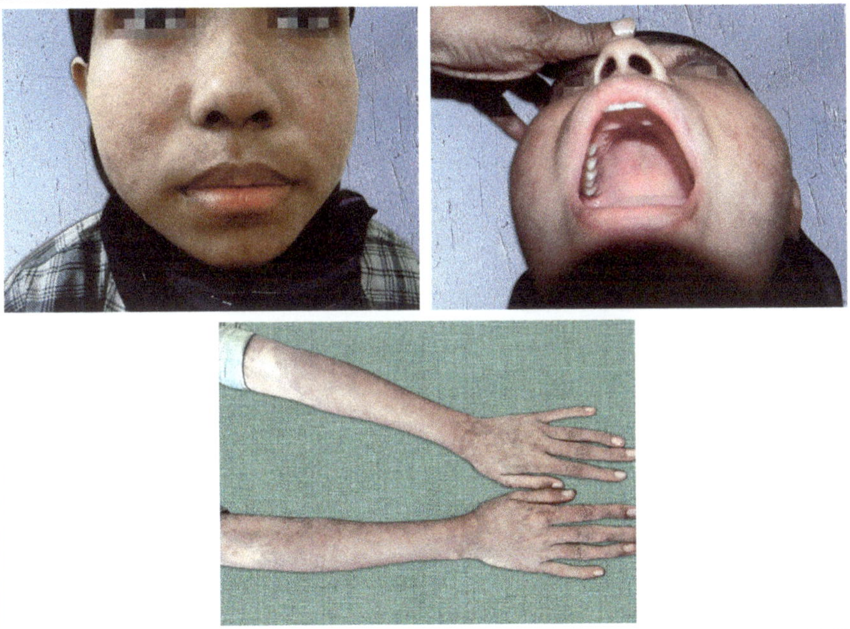

Q. What is the (i) diagnosis and (ii) management?

Answers

i. Systemic lupus erythematosus.

ii. Management

- Referral to rheumatologist
- Strict avoidance of day light
- Oral hydroxychloroquine 200–400 mg by eye monitoring.

Case 124

A 36-year-old male had swelling of left leg (unilaterally) with multiple discharging sinuses (black arrows) liberating pus-containing granules for last 10 years. On palpation the affected area was not tender.

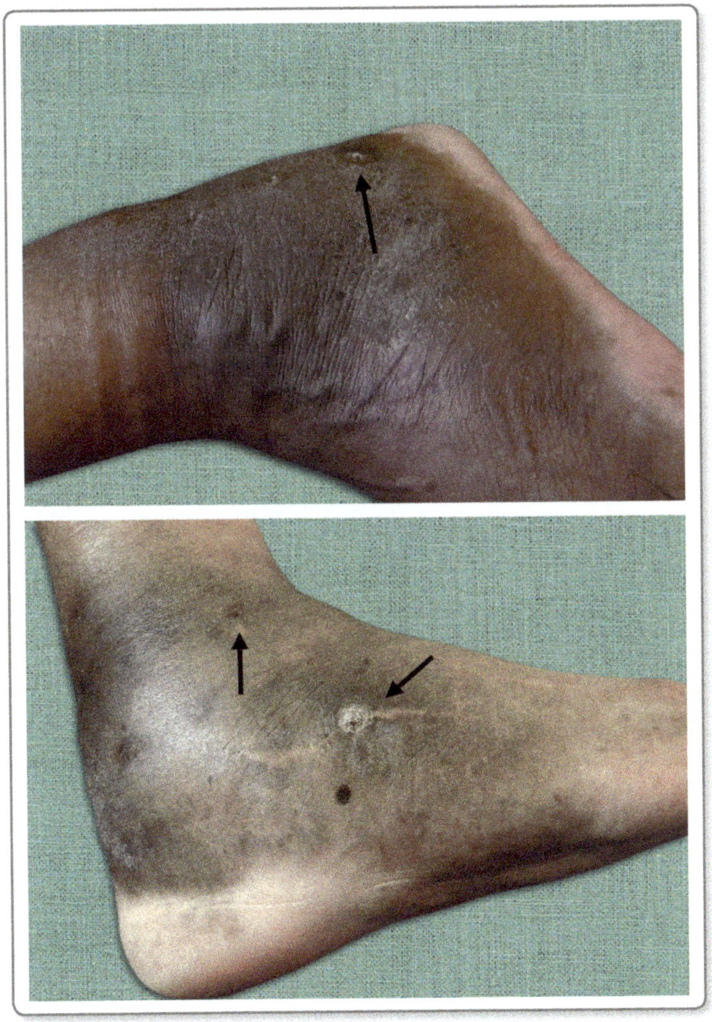

Q. What is the (i) diagnosis and (ii) management?

Answers

i. Mycetoma.

ii. Management

- Confirmation of diagnosis and identification of etiological agents (actinomycetoma or eumycetoma, i.e. true fungi)
- Actinomycetoma: Streptomycin or rifampicin with either cotrimoxazole or dapsone
- Eumycetoma: Ketoconazole or itraconazole.

Case 125

A 28-year-old primigravida at 28 week of gestation had itchy papules, wheals and plaques on her abdomen especially on striae.

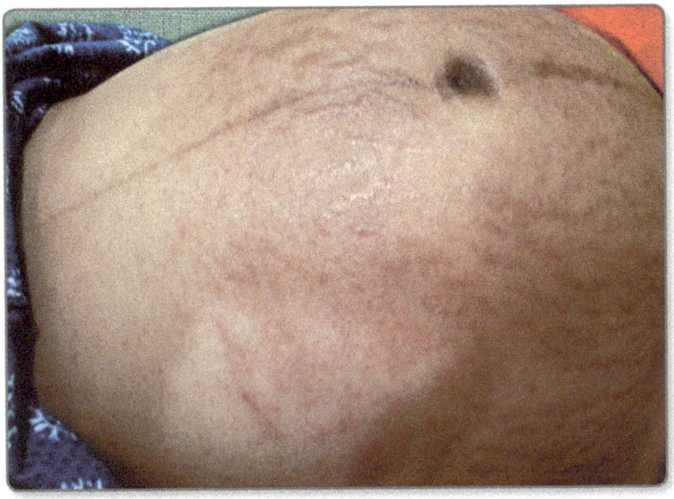

Q. What is the (i) diagnosis and (ii) management?

Answers

i. Pruritic urticarial papules and plaques of pregnancy (PUPPP).

ii. Management
   - Topical corticosteroid
   - Antihistamines.

Case 126

A 34-year-old lady had tiny pigmented macules (white arrows) on face for last 15 years aggravating after sunexposure. She had similar ailment in her mother.

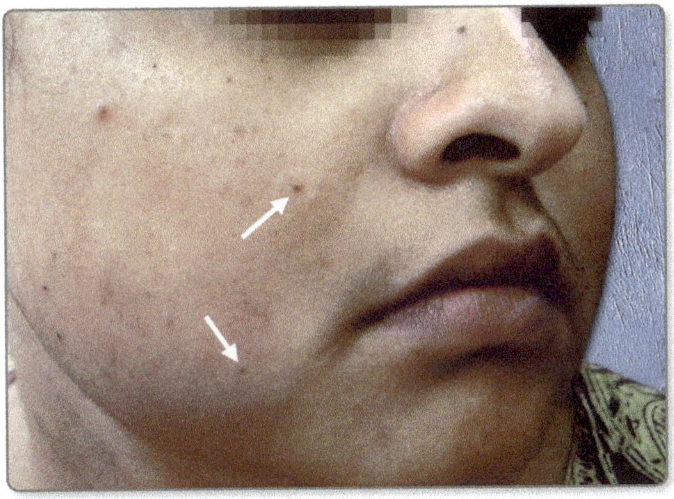

Q. What is the (i) diagnosis and (ii) management?

Answers

i. Freckles.

ii. Management

- Avoidance of daylight by sunscreen, etc.
- Prognosis (incurable nature) to be explained.

Case 127

A 54-year-old male had hyperkeratotic palms and soles for last 10 years with some warty lesions (black arrow). He had also dewdrops like hyper and hypopigmentation over trunk. He had history of ingestion of tubewell water for last 15 years.

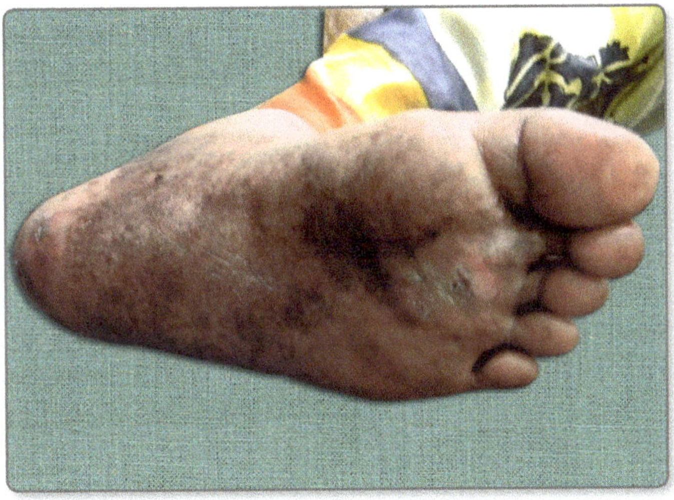

Q. What is the (i) diagnosis and (ii) management?

Answers

i. Arsenic keratosis.

ii. Management

- Avoidance of tubewell water
- Avoid other carcinogens (smoking, sunexposure, etc.)
- Biopsy from the warty lesions to exclude malignancy.

Case 128

A 24-year-old female had recurrent small scaly plaques (black arrow) on limbs and trunk for last 1 year.

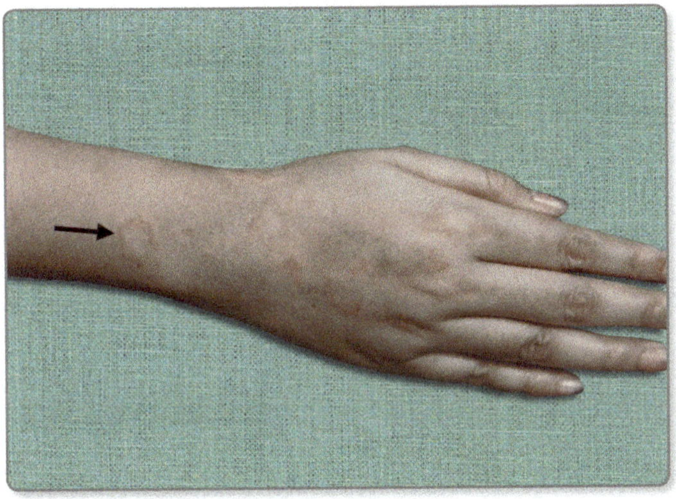

Q. What is the (i) diagnosis and (ii) management?

Answers

i. Small plaque parapsoriasis.
ii. Management
   - Topical steroid
   - PUVA therapy.

Case 129

A 29-year-old male had itchy papules on glans, shaft of the penis for last 2 months. He had history of extra-marital exposure.

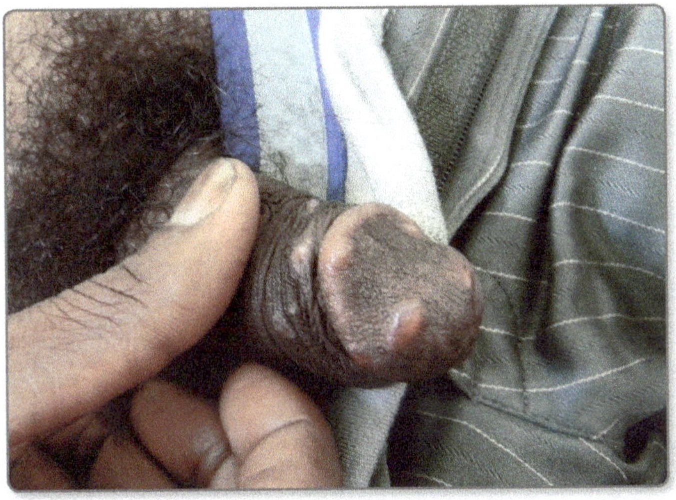

Q. What is the (i) diagnosis and (ii) management?

Answers

i. Scabies (sexually acquired).

ii. Management

- Exclusion of other STDs by proper screening
- Permethrin 5% to apply from neck to feet for 1 night (to repeat once next week).

Case 130

A 21-year-old male had soft swelling one side of left great toe nail for last 3 months which used to bleed often. He had history of trauma 6 months back on that site.

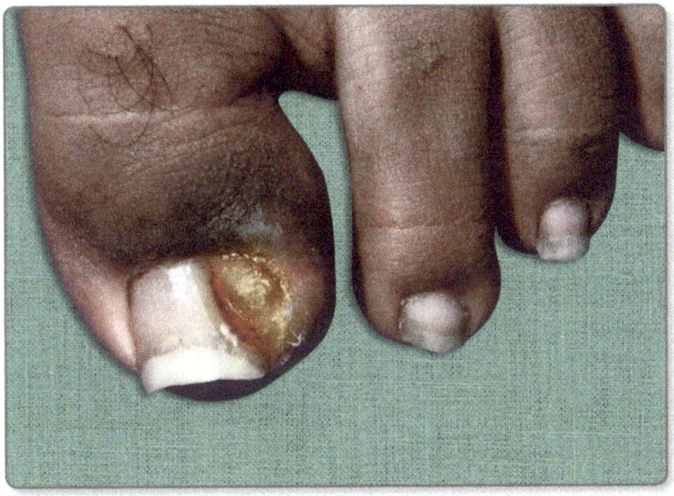

Q. What is the (i) diagnosis and (ii) management?

Answers

i. Granuloma pyogenicum.

ii. Management
- Control of infection
- Chemical cautery or electrocautery or cryotherapy.

Case 131

A 26-year-old male recurrent painful chord-like swelling (black arrow) on legs for last 1 year.

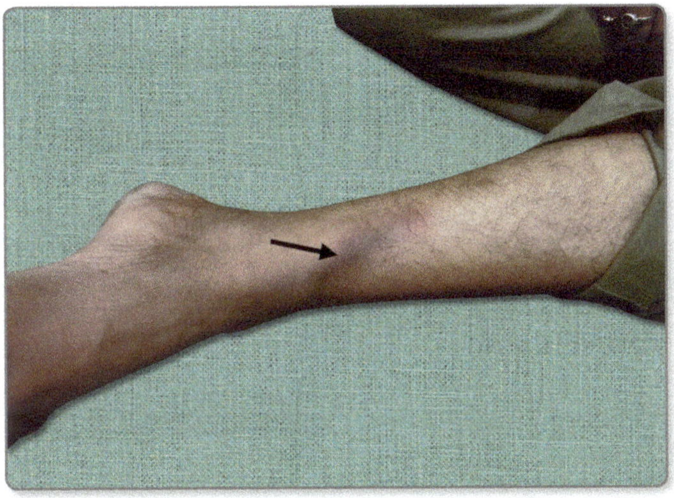

Q. What is the (i) diagnosis and (ii) management?

Answers

i. Recurrent thrombophlebitis.

ii. Management

- Systemic antibiotics
- To search any underlying diseases like pancreatic carcinoma, tuberculosis, etc.

Case 132

A 59-year-old female had recurrent reddish swelling on both eyelids for last 1 year. She had history of taking ACE inhibitor as antihypertensive for last 2 years.

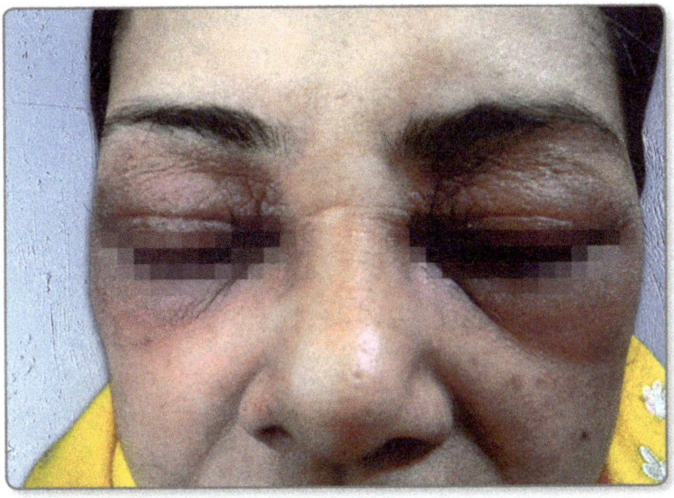

Q. What is the (i) diagnosis and (ii) management?

Answers

i. Acquired angioedema (due to ACE inhibitor).

ii. Management
- Avoidance of ACE inhibitors and also angiotensin-receptor blocking agents (sartan group)
- Oral antihistaminic
- Anti-bradykinin agent.

Case 133

A 43-year-old male had oral erotion, generalized skin eruption (mostly maculopapular) for last 3 weeks with fever. His liver enzymes were quite high. He had history of taking allopurinol for last 2 months for hyperuricemia.

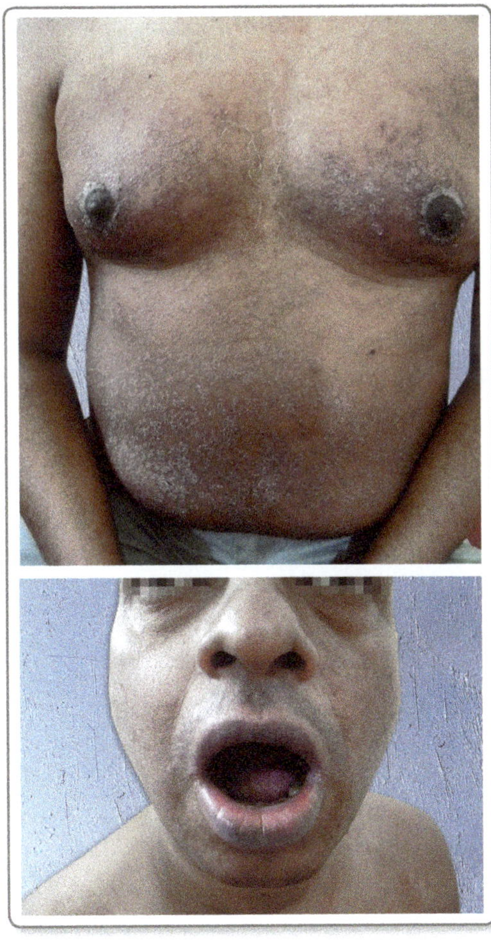

Q. What is the (i) diagnosis and (ii) management?

Answers

i. Drug hypersensitivity syndrome (DHS) (due to allopurinol).

iii Management

- Immediate withdrawal of allopurinol
- Admission under dermatologist and internist
- Screening, monitoring and supporting treatment of systemic involvement
- Oral corticosteroid by monitoring.

Case 134

A 64-year-old male had chronic dry eczematous lesions on lower legs for last 6 months being aggravated in winter.

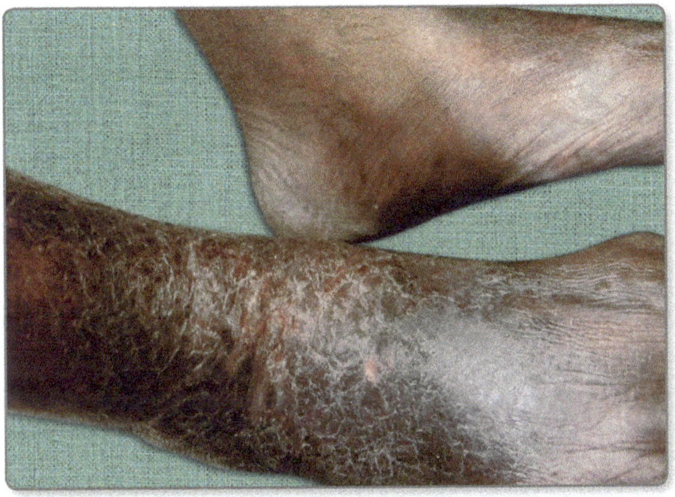

Q. What is the (i) diagnosis and (ii) management?

Answers

i. Asteatotic eczema.
ii. Management
   - Avoidance of soap
   - Screening for diabetes and hypothyroid
   - Topical emollient (containing urea, etc.)
   - Topical steroid in ointment
   - Oral antihistamines.

Case 135

A 45-year-old female had swelling, puffiness and nodules on ear lobules, face and different area of trunk. The lesions were juicy, shiny, and soft.

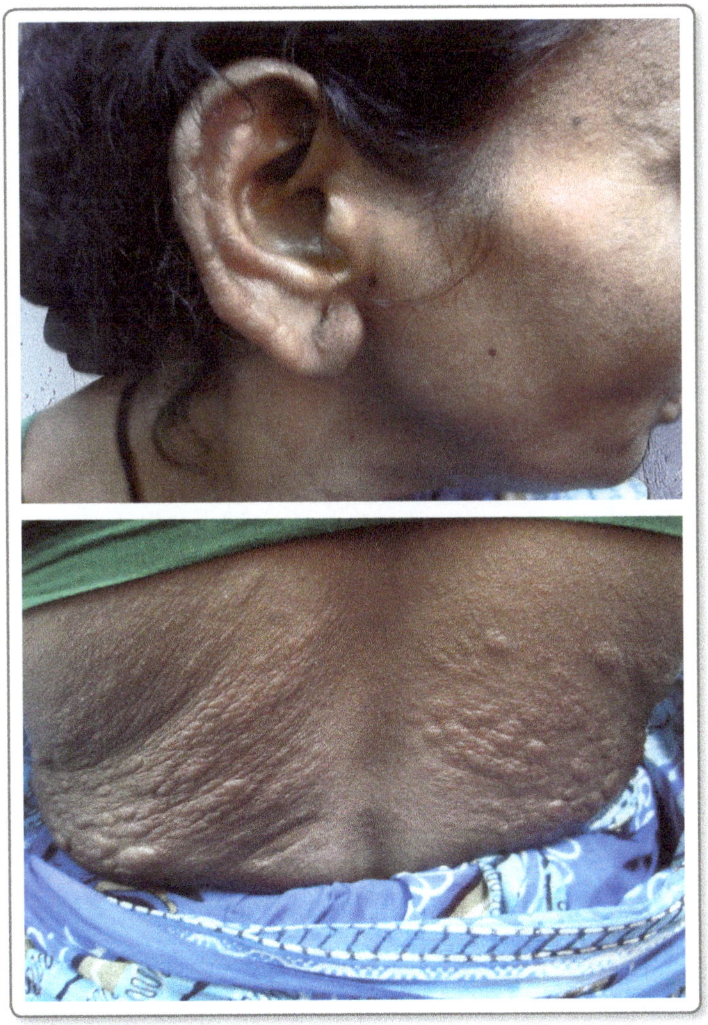

Q. What is the (i) diagnosis and (ii) management?

Answers

i. Lepromatous leprosy.

ii. Management

- Dapsone 100 mg daily
- Clofazimine 100 mg on alternate day, and 300 mg once monthly
- Rifampicin 600 mg once monthly in empty stomach (supervised).

Case 136

A 47-year-old female had mutiple skin-colored nodules on axillae and neck for last 3 years. She had history of diabetes for last 10 years.

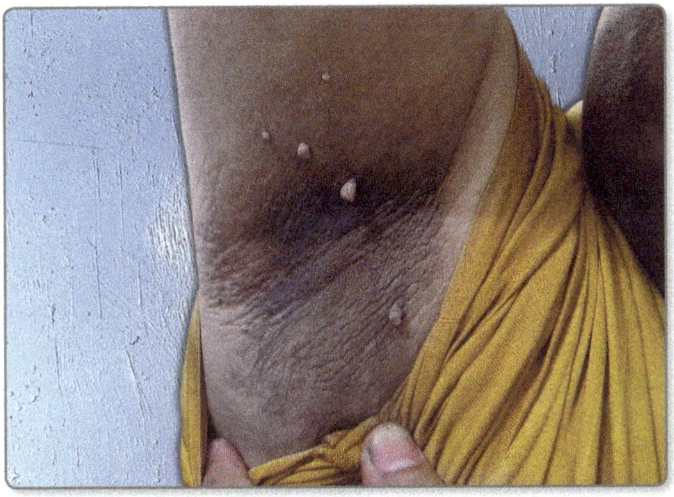

Q. What is the (i) diagnosis and (ii) management?

Answers

i. Acrochordon (skin tags).

ii. Management
   - Control of diabetes
   - Electrocautery or cryotherapy.

Case 137

A 21-year-old female had highly pruritic hyperkeratotic papules or nodules on limbs and trunk for last 2 years.

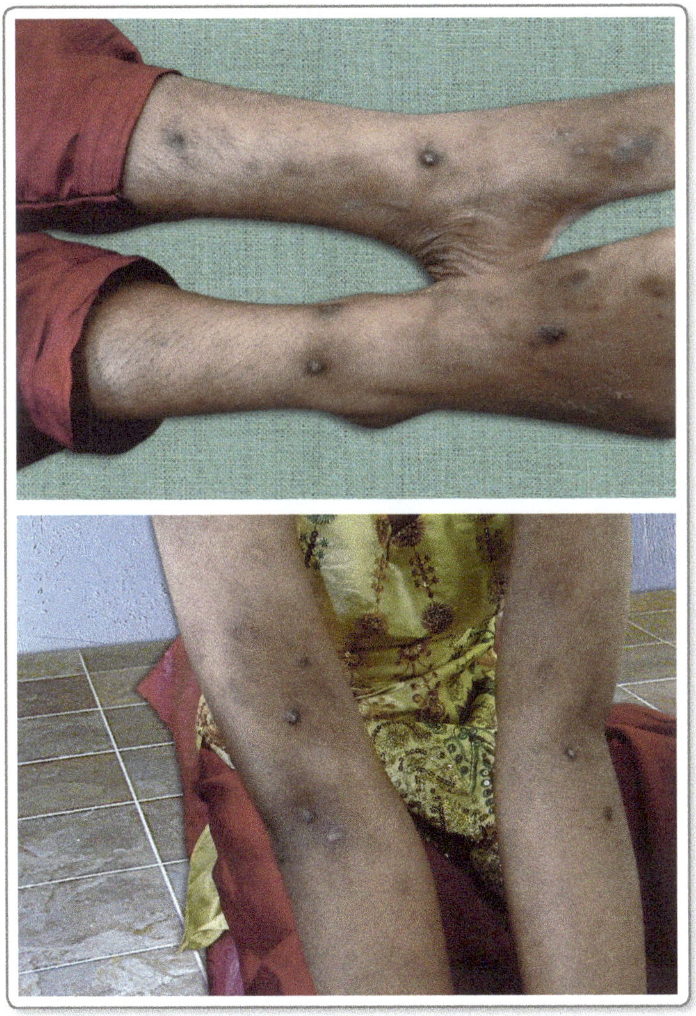

Q. What is the (i) diagnosis and (ii) management?

Answers

i. Prurigo nodularis.
ii. Management
   - Topical super potent corticosteroid
   - Oral antihistaminic.

Case 138

A 18-year-old male had linear depressed pigmented lesion (black arrow) on central forehead for last 3 years.

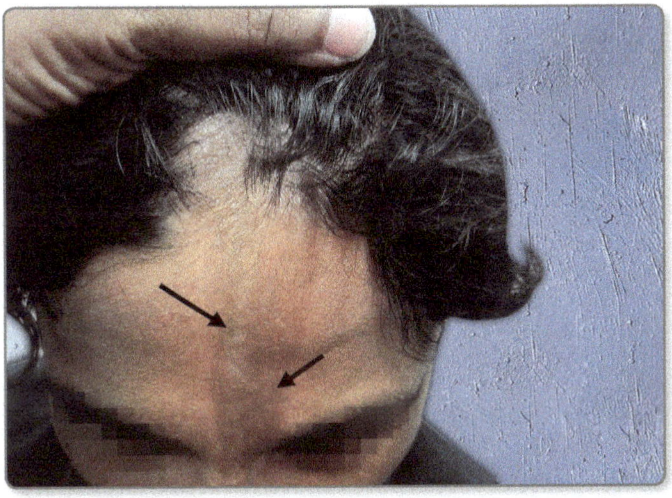

Q. What is the (i) diagnosis and (ii) management?

Answers

i. Linear morphea (localized scleroderma).
ii. Management
- Topical vitamin D analog
- Topical mid-potent steroid.

Case 139

A 10-year-old boy had recurrent itchy eczematous lesions on limbs and trunk predominately affecting flexors since last 5 years. He had also history of bronchial asthma.

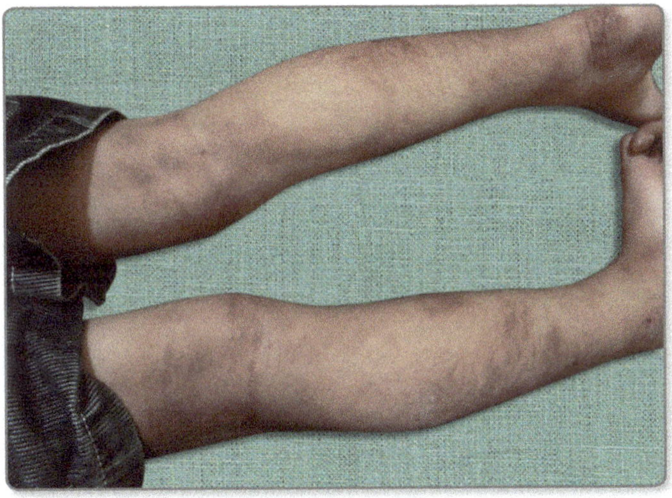

Q. What is the (i) diagnosis and (ii) management?

Answers

i. Atopic dermatitis.

ii. Management
- Avoidance of triggering factors (dust mite, pollens, etc.)
- Topical emollients liberally
- Topical low potent steroid or tacrolimus/pimecrolimus
- Oral antihistamines.

Case 140

A 51-year-old male had pruritic hives mostly in linear configuration especially after stroking.

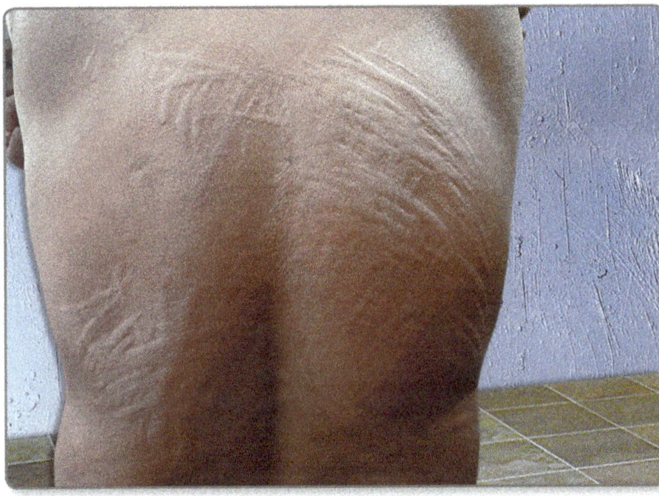

Q. What is the (i) diagnosis and (ii) management?

Answers

i. Dermographism (symptomatic).

ii. Management

- Avoidance of triggering factors (especially stroking, etc.)
- Oral antihistaminic.

Case 141

A 29-year-old male had eruption on both groin for last 6 months. He had applied topical antifungal and corticosteroid combination for last 3 months. At the beginning some suppression of the lesion occurred but later the eruption continued to spread. On examination, the lesion had annular border (arrow) and central clearing with hypopigmentation at some area.

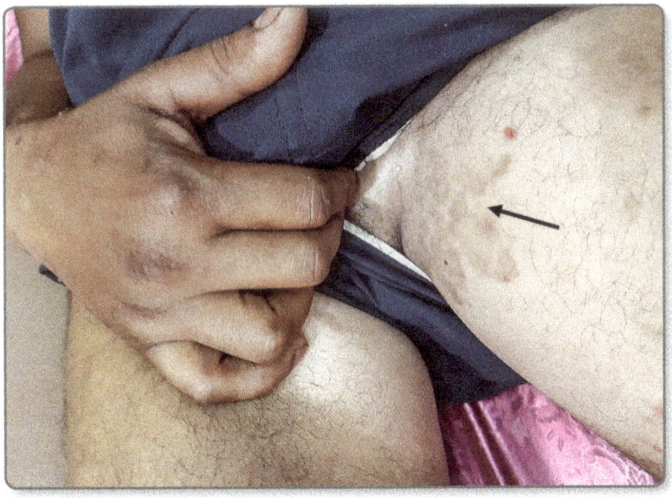

Q. What is the (i) diagnosis and (ii) management?

Answers

i. Tinea cruris with steroid-modification.

ii. Management

- Strict avoidance of topical corticosteroids
- Oral terbinafine 250 OD for 15 days
  or, oral fluconazole 150 mg once/week for 4 weeks
  or, oral itraconazole 100 mg BD for 14 days
- Topical terbinafine, sertaconazole, luliconazole, or amorolfine daily for 4 weeks.

Case 142

A 7-year-old boy had itchy warty lesions on left hand, forearm and arm since birth which had been slowly increasing as age being advanced.

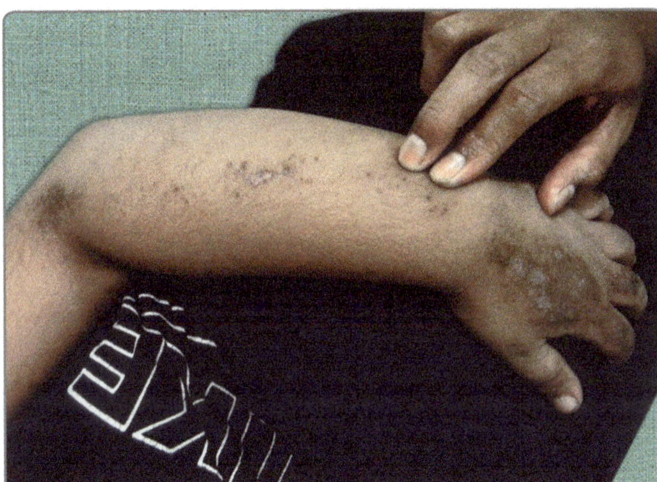

Q. What is the (i) diagnosis and (ii) management?

Answers

i. Linear epidermal nevus.

ii. Management
   - Prognosis to be discussed
   - Electrocautery or cryotherapy may be tried.

Case 143

A 72-year-old male had itching and pain with redness on feet in deep winter especially when exposed to cold water.

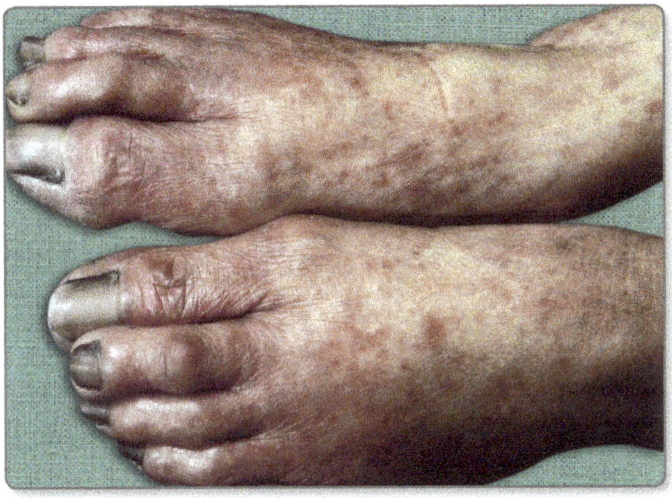

Q. What is the (i) diagnosis and (ii) management?

Answers

i. Chilblain.

ii. Management
   - Avoidance of cold exposure
   - Use of socks
   - Topical steroid.

Case 144

A 51-year-old female had acute swelling with pain on corner of right thumb nail for last 1 week. She was a known diabetic.

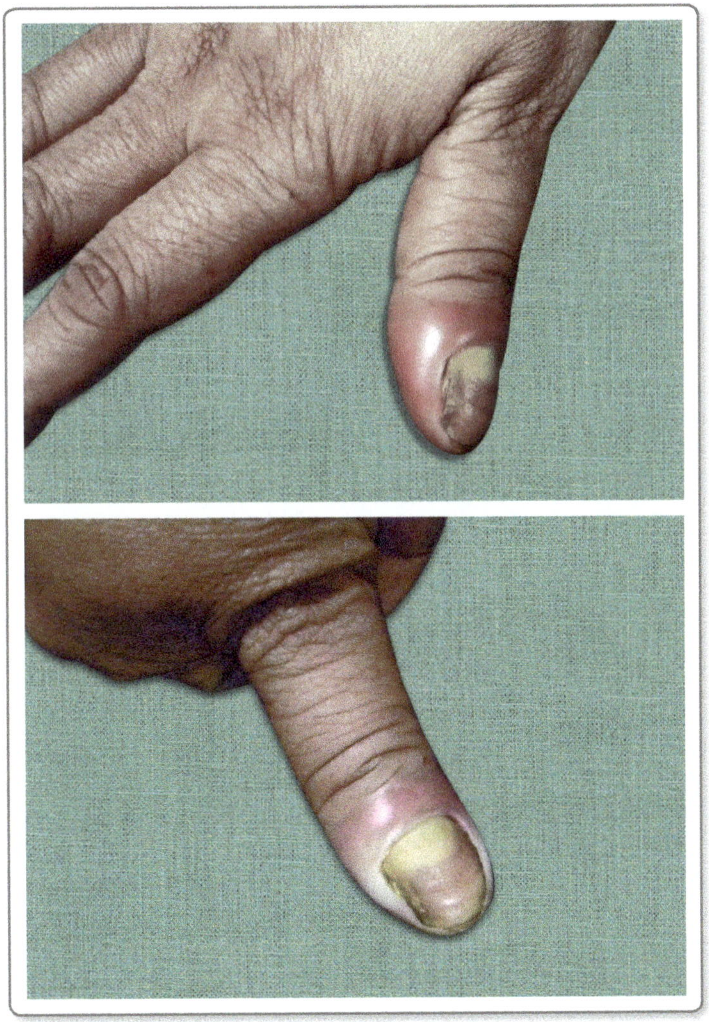

Q. What is the (i) diagnosis and (ii) management?

Answers

i. Acute paronychia.

ii. Management
   - Referral to surgeon
   - Oral or injectable antibioitic
   - Incision and drainage.

Case 145

A 34-year-old male had thick warty lesion on side and underneath the nail of right middle finger.

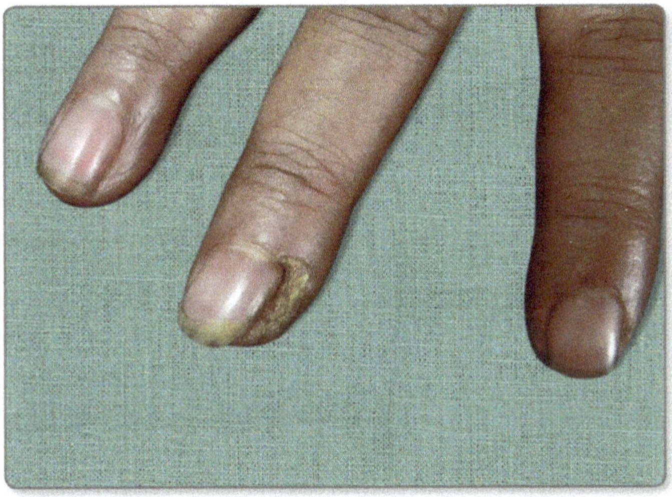

Q. What is the (i) diagnosis and (ii) management?

Answers

i. Periungual verruca (wart).

ii. Management

- Chemical cautery
  or
  Electrocautery
  or
  Cryotherapy.

Case 146

A 39-year-old male had unilateral itchy scaly eruption on left sole with involvement of first interdigital web (arrow) space for last 3 months.

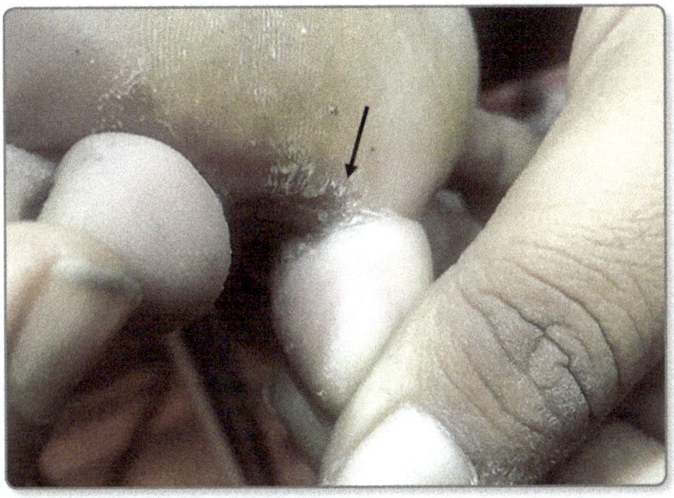

Q. What is the (i) diagnosis and (ii) management?

Answers

i. Tinea pedis.

ii. Management

- Oral terbinafine 250 OD for 15 days
  or, oral fluconazole 150 mg once/week for 4 weeks
  or, oral itraconazole 100 mg BD for 14 days
- Topical terbinafine, sertaconazole, luliconazole or amorolfine daily for 4 weeks.

Case 147

A 17-year-old female had chronic inflammatory pustules on arms and trunk for last 8 months, which aggravated during humid season. There were no comedones among the lesions.

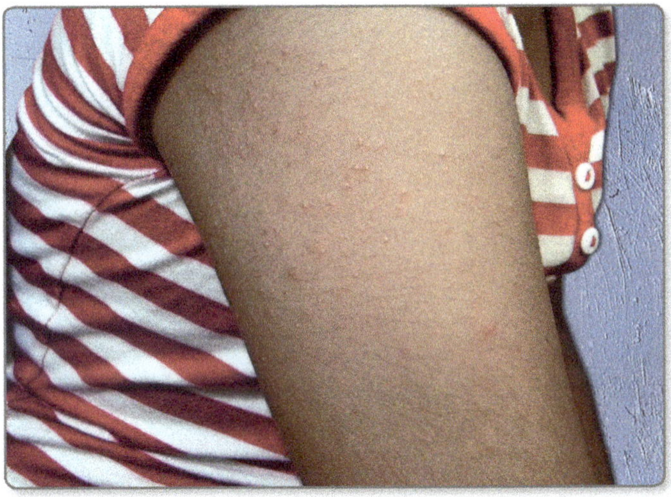

Q. What is the (i) diagnosis and (ii) management?

Answers

i. Pityrosporum folliculitis.

ii Management

- Topical antifungal (like miconazole gel)
- Oral antifungal, if refractory.

Case 148

A 45-year-old lady had acute eczematous eruption along hair margin for last 2 weeks. She had history of application of black mehndi on hair during last few months.

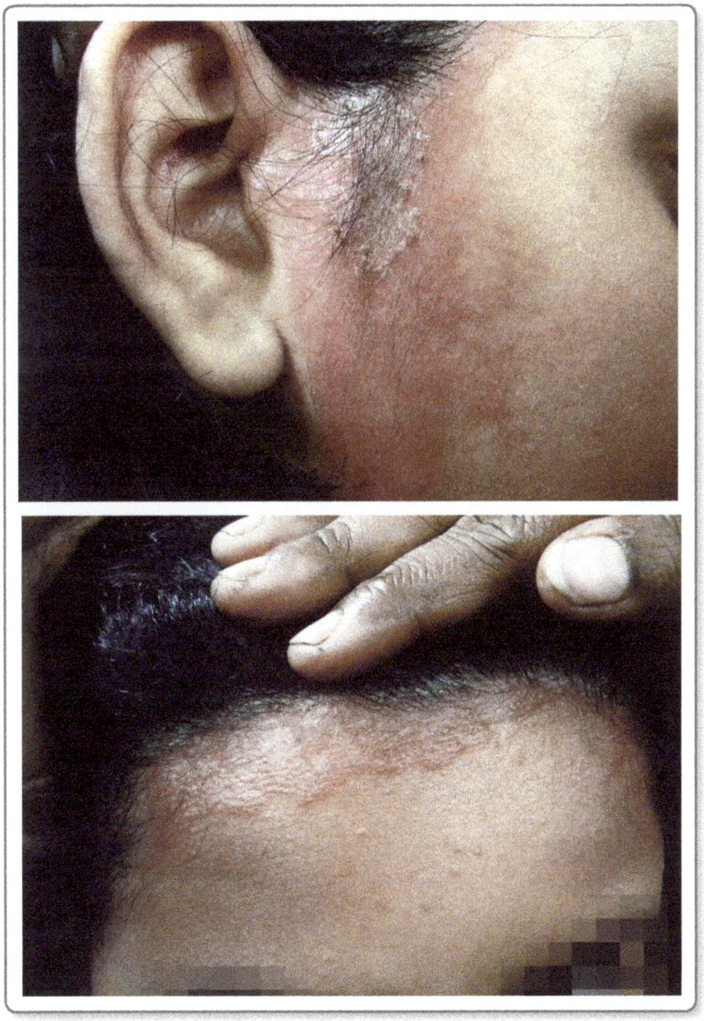

Q. What is the (i) diagnosis and (ii) management?

Answers

i. Allergic contact dermatitis from PPD (in hair dye).

ii. Management

  a. Strict avoidance of any PPD-containing dye
  b. Topical mometasone lotion
  c. Oral antihistamines.

Case 149

A 9-year-old male had generalized itching mostly aggravated during night for last 4 weeks. He showed excoriated papules and vesicle at interdigital area and periumbilical area and he has similar episodes in family members.

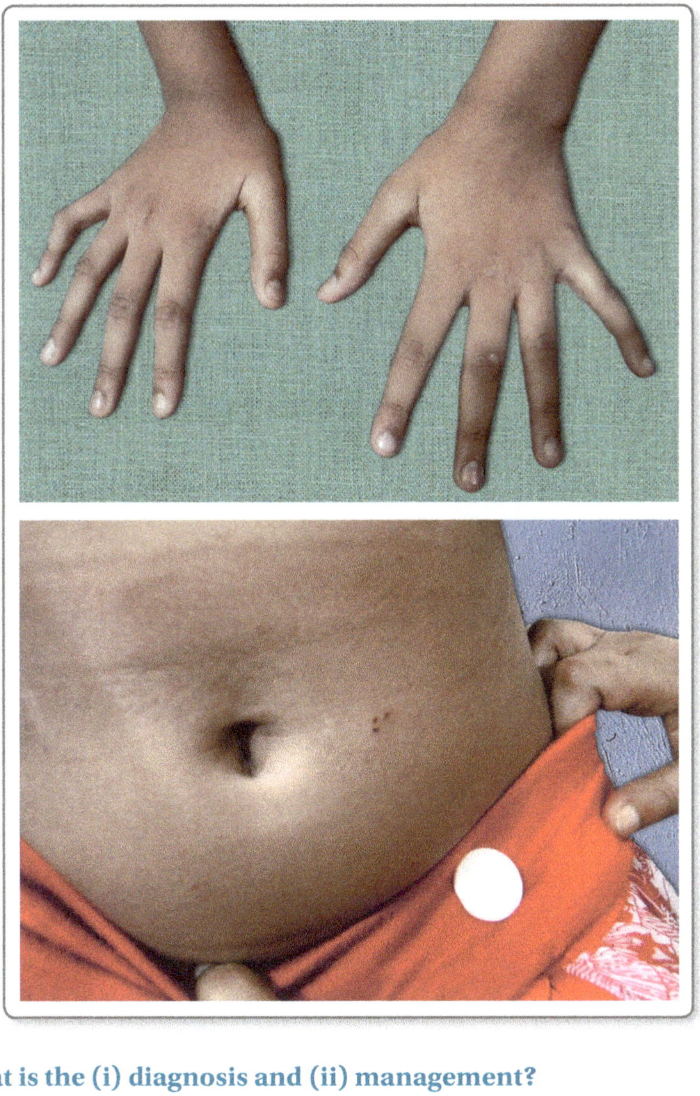

Q. What is the (i) diagnosis and (ii) management?

Answers

i. Scabies.

ii. Management

- Permethrin 5% cream from neck to feet at one night to be repeated next week once
- Hot washing of clothes and fomites
- Oral antihistamines
- Treatment of family members.

Case 150

A 43-year-old lady had recurrent swelling and pain on right middle finger nail for 3 months. She was treated with antibiotics but had only temporary relief.

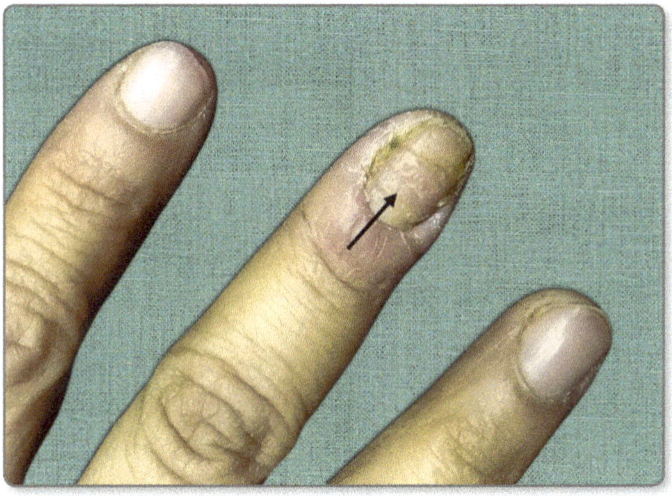

Q. What is the (i) diagnosis and (ii) management?

Answers

i. Chronic paronychia.

ii. Management

- Oral fluconazole 150 mg once/week for 4 weeks
  or, oral itraconazole 100 mg BD for 14 days
- Topical clotrimazole, sertaconazole, luliconazole or amorolfine daily for 4 weeks.

Case 151

A 63-year-old male had thick hyperkeratotic scaly lesions on scalp for last 5 years aggravating during winter. The lesions had a well-defined margin along the frontal hairline. His nails showed pitting.

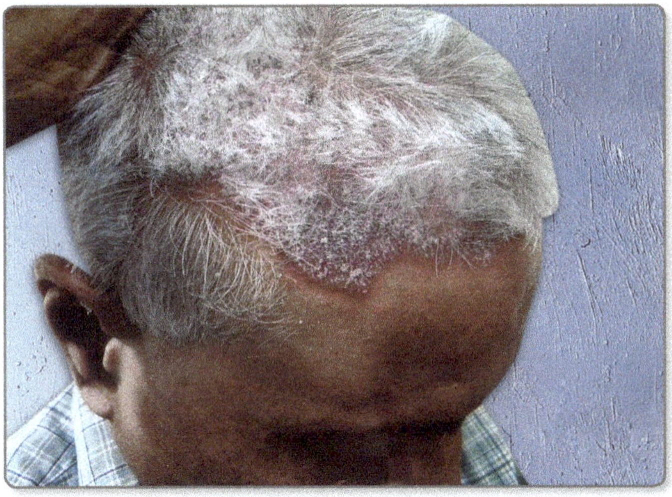

Q. What is the (i) diagnosis and (ii) management?

Answers

i. Psoriasis.
ii. Management
- Tar shampoo
- Topical steroid plus salicylic acid 3–6% lotion
- PUVA, if refractory.

Index

D

E

O

P

T

U

V

W

X

Y

Z

EU GSPR Authorised Reprsentative
Logos Europe, 9 rue Nicolas Poussin
1700, La Rochelle, France
Phone: +33 (0) 6 67 93 73 78
E-mail: contact@logoseurope.eu

www.ingramcontent.com/pod-product-compliance
Ingram Content Group UK Ltd.
Pitfield, Milton Keynes, MK11 3LW, UK
UKHW061546190726
13845UKWH00030B/1042

* 9 7 8 9 3 5 2 7 0 4 9 2 7 *